Swiss Ball

For Strength, Tone, and Posture

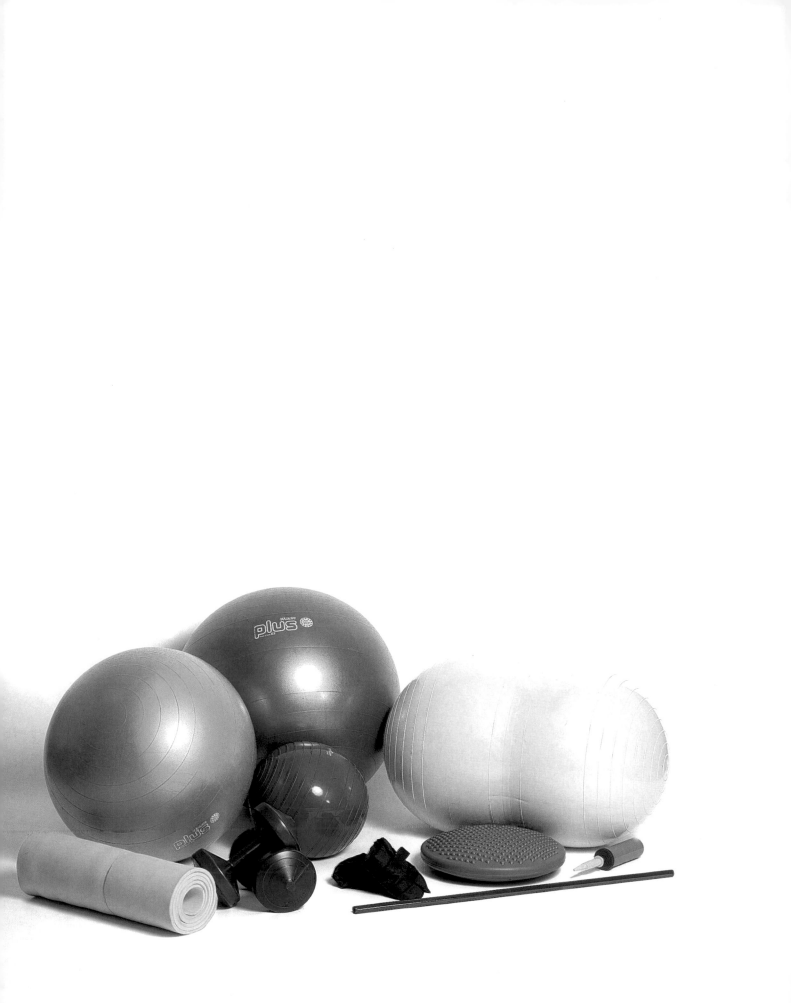

Swiss Ball

For Strength, Tone, and Posture

Maureen Flett

PRC

Produced 2003 by

PRC Publishing Limited

The Chrysalis Building

Bramley Road, London W10 6SP

An imprint of **Chrysalis** Books Group plc

This edition published 2004

Distributed in the U.S. and Canada by:

Sterling Publishing Co., Inc.

387 Park Avenue South

New York, NY 10016

ISBN 1 85648 663-X

Printed and bound in Malaysia

ACKNOWLEDGMENTS

The publisher wishes to thank Simon Clay for taking all the photography in this book,
including the photographs on the front and back covers. All photography is copyright © PRC Publishing 2003.
All enquiries regarding the images should be referred to Chrysalis Images.

All products used in this book are available from www.thesportsphysio.com

SAFETY NOTE

The exercises are for information only and are not intended to replace
appropriate advice from a qualified practitioner. Any person suffering from conditions
requiring medical attention should consult a qualified medical practitioner
before undertaking any exercises from this book.

Contents

Introduction

History of the Swiss Ball

The Swiss Ball was developed in 1963 by Italian plastics manufacturer Aquilino Cosani, who pioneered a unique process for molding large, colorful balls, which could be filled with air. Mary Quinton, a British physiotherapist working in Switzerland, began using these balls in treatment programs for newborns and infants and subsequently introduced them to the UK.

Dr. Susan Klein-Vogelbach, a founding director of a physical therapy school in Basel, Switzerland, was the first to use these balls with adults who had orthopedic or other medical problems.

Although the balls are Italian in origin, American physical therapists first witnessed their use in Switzerland, and this was how the term "Swiss Ball" was born. It was introduced to the United States in 1989 by Joanne Posner-Mayer, and physical therapists began using the balls for neurological, orthopedic, and fitness programs.

The Swiss ball is now known by many names including, Gym Ball, Body Ball, or Gymnastic Ball, and is widely employed in fitness and training programs for many elite athletes and teams.

Benefits of using a Swiss Ball

Low cost

Swiss Balls provide training without the use of expensive equipment or the need to go to a gym. They are easily portable, which ensures you can take your "gym" with you no matter where you are.

Coordination and proprioception are developed at the same time

The ball provides an unstable base, allowing more than one muscle group to be active at any one time. The brain and muscles have to concentrate on balance as well as the exercise being performed.

Although this book is broken down into sections relating to areas of the body, it is virtually impossible to only train one muscle group while using the ball.

Throughout this book, the word proprioception will be mentioned many times, but what does it mean? For a muscle to perform an activity, a signal has to be sent from the muscle to the brain and back again. This happens very quickly. Specialized nerve endings, located in muscles and tendons, transmit information that is used to control the action of a limb or muscle. These nerve endings are called proprioceptors.

To find out how good your proprioception is, try standing on one leg, the foot on the floor should not wobble and you should be able to maintain balance for quite a period of time. Now close your eyes and if your proprioception is good, you should still be able to keep balance without wobbling. Training proprioception will improve your balance and coordination.

Multifunctional

We need to remember that muscles always work in pairs. For example, when the biceps in front of the upper arm are lifting the forearm, the triceps at the back of the upper arm are lengthening to control the movement and vice versa, replicating the type of actions needed for sporting or everyday activity. The introduction to the Core Stability section on page 22 goes into greater detail on this subject.

Using a Swiss Ball adds a different dimension to your exercise regime and complements many other training programs. You do not have to be an elite athlete to benefit from training with the exercise ball. Many back pain sufferers find the ball invaluable in rehabilitation. Senior citizens and pregnant women like using the exercise ball as it provides a more comfortable environment.

What results can you expect from using an exercise ball?

- Improved posture
- Enhanced muscle tone
- Greater strength and control of the active and stabilizing muscle groups
- Increased agility and speed
- Reduced risk of injury

The terminology of the anatomy and muscle groups being worked in each section has been kept to a basic level. It is outside the remit of this book to go into great anatomical detail or the training of certain muscle groups for specific purposes.

Each section of the book is broken down into color coded basic, intermediate, and advanced sections. The basic sections concentrate on correcting the posture and alignment and encouraging the sense of balance. The medicine ball and stability cushion are introduced in the intermediate sections to add a strengthening aspect to the exercises and further work the sense of balance. Weights are introduced into the advanced section to strengthen particular muscle groups, making the exercises more sports specific.

Safety Precautions

Before commencing any exercise with the ball, please ensure you have checked the following:

Ball inflation: Make sure you have the right size ball. Seated on the ball, your hips should be level or slightly higher than your knees with your feet flat on the floor. Ensure that the ball is correctly inflated. Please follow the manufacturer's instructions.

Ball storage: Follow the manufacturer's instructions and do not store the balls near heat sources or in very cold temperatures as this could affect the expansion properties of the material.

Exercise area: Give yourself plenty of free space to perform the exercises. Make sure the floor is non-slip and free from any debris such as grit or splinters, which may damage or puncture the ball.

Clothing: Do not wear clothing, which is slippery or too baggy, this will result in lack of grip and could cause you to fall from the ball. If using footwear, wear something that allows you to grip and is not too heavy or chunky.

Weights: When progressing to the intermediate and advanced sections, many of the exercises will use weights, medicine balls, etc. Never use any weight that you cannot lift comfortably, remember that the ball provides an unstable base and this will make lifting the weight much more difficult.

Ensure all equipment is in good working order: Always use an antiburst ball, which is designed to take up to at least 600lb (300kg) and never let the combined weight of the equipment and your body exceed that of the manufacturer's recommendations.

Exercise safety: The layout of this book is provided for your safety, work from basic to intermediate and then to advanced, only progressing onto the next stage when the exercise becomes easy and your body is not struggling to keep the ball steady. For some of the intermediate and advanced exercises, it would be wise to have a friend or partner to assist. Do not attempt any exercise that you are unsure of. Do not exercise within half an hour of a meal and two hours of a heavy meal.

Health: If you are not used to exercising or have a medical condition, please check with your physician / doctor before commencing any form of exercise.

Equipment

For the exercises in this book you will require the following equipment, although for the basic exercises an exercise ball will suffice.

Exercise ball: Ensure it is the correct size and of antiburst quality.

Physio Roll*: Similar to the ball, but shaped like a peanut for added stability. Ideal if you have disabilities or balance problems.

Stability Cushion*: A circular PVC cushion that can be inflated with air.

Exercise mat

Pole: Needs to be 4–5 ft (1.2m) in length; a bamboo cane will do.

Medicine ball: A specially weighted exercise ball ranging from 2–11 lb (1–5kg). Ensure you stay within your comfortable lifting range.

Resistive therapy band: A stretchy band, with six or eight levels of resistance, often identified by color.

Ankle weights: The wrap around type is best with adjustable weight levels.

Set of dumbbells: Make sure they are within your comfortable lifting range.

Pump: Needed to blow up the ball. The type of pump required will depend on the manufacturer of the ball.

* Registered trademark of Ledraplastic Spa., Italy.

How to choose the correct size of ball

Sizing is generally based on your height. When seated on a ball, your hips should be slightly higher than your knees and your feet should be flat on the floor.

As a rule, the length of your arm from shoulder to fingertip is a very good guide to finding the right size of ball.

Length of arm	Ball size required
22–25½in (56–65cm)	21½in (55cm) diameter
26–31½in (66–80cm)	25½in (65cm) diameter
31⅞–35½in (81–90cm)	29½in (75cm) diameter
35½in+ (90cm+)	33½in (85cm) diameter

Please note that these sizes apply only to the Gymnic range of exercise balls, which do inflate to their published diameter and should not be applied to any other make of ball. Each manufacturer will provide their sizing instructions.

How to inflate the ball

This will depend greatly on the manufacturer and their advice should be followed at all times. Always use a hand-operated pump, never use an electric compressor.

Neutral Alignment and Posture

For the exercises contained in this book to work effectively, it is vitally important that you learn how to obtain neutral alignment.

Neutral alignment can be simplified into thinking of your body as a series of building blocks.

- Head
- Shoulders
- Rib cage
- Pelvis
- Legs

These blocks should all be stacked neatly on top of each other, in order for the body to function in the correct way.

Stand side on to a full length mirror, you should be able to draw an imaginary straight line down your side through your ears, shoulders, elbows, hips, knees, and ankle. Any deviation from this is out of alignment and needs work.

Breathing is just as important during exercise and needs to be coordinated with each movement that you do.

- Breathe in before a movement
- Breathe out during the movement.

Many people during this type of exercise have a habit of holding their breath, not only is this bad for the oxygen content of the blood but can lead to heart and lung complications.

Unfortunately, as a result of our sedentary lifestyles and poor posture, most of us breathe using our stomach muscles and so do not use the lungs to their full capacity.

Try the following exercise. Get yourself a long scarf or towel and wrap it around your rib cage so that the loose ends are crossed over in the middle of your chest. Hold on to either end of the scarf or towel to keep it tight and breathe in, as you breathe in try to force your ribs outward against the towel in all directions, forward, backward, and sideways. Once you have the general idea, practice doing these simple alignment exercises and controlling your breathing at the same time, just as though you still have the towel or scarf around your chest. Follow the next three exercises carefully. Before commencing any work on the ball you must be happy that you can attain a neutral spine in all of the three positions.

Finding Neutral—Supine

Level: All

Before commencing any exercise using the gym ball, it is vitally important to ensure that you are able to find the following neutral positions.

These positions ensure effectiveness and safety of the exercise as well as activating the lower abdominal and pelvic stabilizing muscles, which form a protective and supportive girdle to the lumbar spine.

Lay on the exercise mat, with your knees bent and feet placed flat on the floor.

Pull the navel backward toward the floor to tighten the lower abdominal muscles. (If you are unsure that these muscles are being activated, press your fingers just above the pelvic bones. You will feel the deeper muscles tighten as you pull the stomach muscles in).

The back must not arch or hollow (you should not be able to put your hand between your back and the floor). Breathing should be relaxed and steady filling the whole of the rib cage.

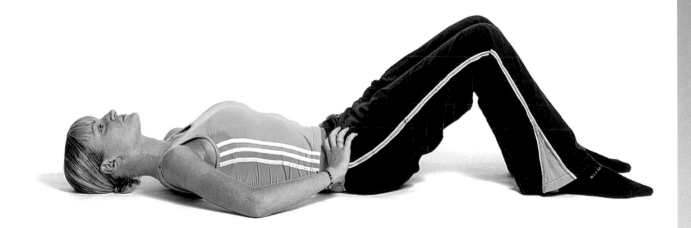

Sitting Alignment

Level: All

Sit on the ball with your back straight. Feet are shoulder
width apart. Tighten your lower abdominal muscles (if
you are unsure, place fingers just above ridge of pelvis
and feel deeper muscles activate as you pull the navel
backward toward the spine). Relax your shoulders and
gently squeeze your shoulder blades together to prevent
your shoulders from rounding.

Breathing should be slow and steady into the rib cage
(the stomach muscles should not move when breathing).

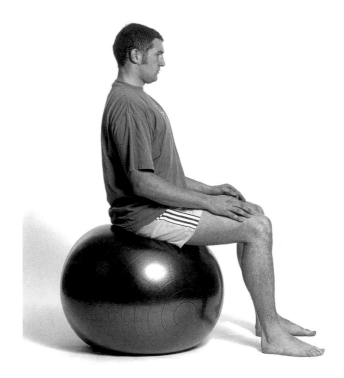

Correct position.

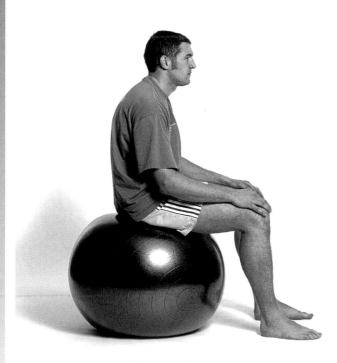

Wrong position.

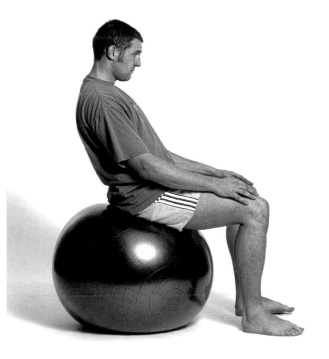

Wrong position.

Finding Neutral—Prone

Level: All

Kneel with the ball under your abdomen. Roll forward until the ball is under your knees or shins.

Pull in the stomach muscles and tighten the buttock muscles (gluteals) so that your spine becomes straight.

Try to hold this position for a while, until you are sure that you can master this quickly and easily.

During all exercises the spine remains level (like a table top) and should not be allowed to sag or arch.

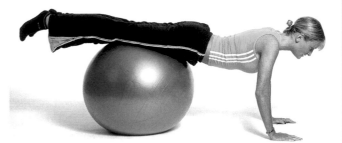

Wrong position.

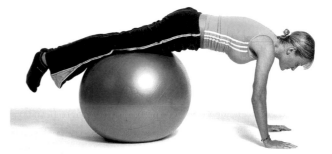

Wrong position.

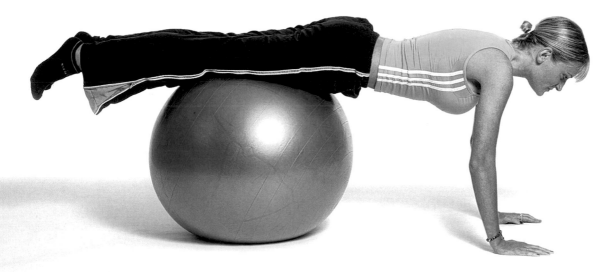

Correct position.

Warm Up and Cool Down

Warming up before any exercise is important because it:

- Prepares the muscles and joints for the activity ahead
- Reduces the risk of injury
- Encourages circulation to the muscles, heart, and lungs
- Allows you to get into the right frame of mind

A warm-up session should last at least 15–20 minutes and each stretch should be gentle but strong, lasting about 10–15 seconds with no pain or burning sensations.

Allow yourself to concentrate on your breathing technique during this warm-up activity. Use the same stretches in this section to cool down after your exercise session to loosen any muscles that may feel tightened or cramped.

Spine Stretch—Forward bending (flexion)
Level: All

During everyday activity and especially when seated for long periods of time, the bones of the spine (vertebrae) become compressed, squashing down on the discs, resulting in stiffness, restricted movement, and backache. Using the ball to support the spine, it is easy to "unlock" this stiffness.

Kneeling with the ball in front, roll forward so that the ball is under your abdomen.

Relax in this position for about 30 seconds, allowing your body to mold itself over the ball. Some people also find it helpful to gently rock back and forth on the ball.

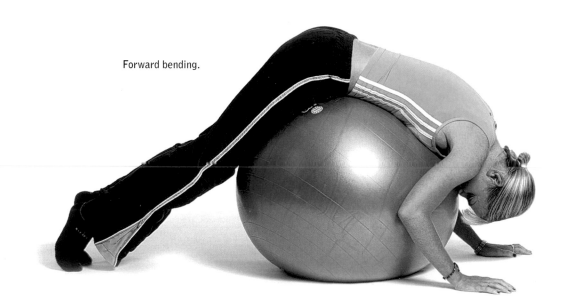

Forward bending.

Spine Stretch—Bending Backward (extension)

Sit on the ball and roll forward so that it is under your lower back.

Gently lower yourself backward over the ball. Do not let your neck bend too far (use a hand to support your head if you have a neck problem).

Hold this position, again rocking if needed, for about 30 seconds.

Gently lower yourself backward over the ball.

Shoulder Stretch

Level: All

This exercise stretches the muscles in the front of the shoulder and chest.

Kneel on the floor or exercise mat with the ball out in front of your head.

Place one hand on the ball and then the other. Allow your body to relax downward so that your can feel a stretch in the front of the shoulder.

Hold for 10–15 seconds, release and repeat three or four times.

Allow your body to relax toward the floor.

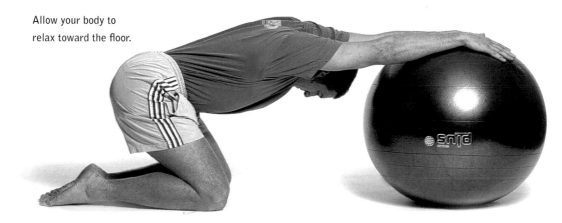

Piriformis Stretch

Level: All

The piriformis is a very small muscle that lies deep underneath the gluteals and is attached to the pelvis and top of the leg. Its job is to turn out the thigh and stop the knee from hanging inward.

This muscle often becomes over tense, leading to lack of mobility in the hip and in some cases compressing the sciatic nerve, which runs under or through it, resulting in pain in the lower back and down the leg (sciatica), often mistaken for disc problems.

Lie on the floor or exercise mat with your left heel on the ball and bring your right leg up to rest your ankle across your left knee.

Tighten your lower abdominal muscles and using your left foot, pull the ball toward your pelvis so that a pull is felt in the gluteal muscles of the right side.

Hold for 15 seconds, keeping the ball as steady as possible and return to the start position. Repeat using the opposite leg.

Limit this exercise to four repetitions on each side.

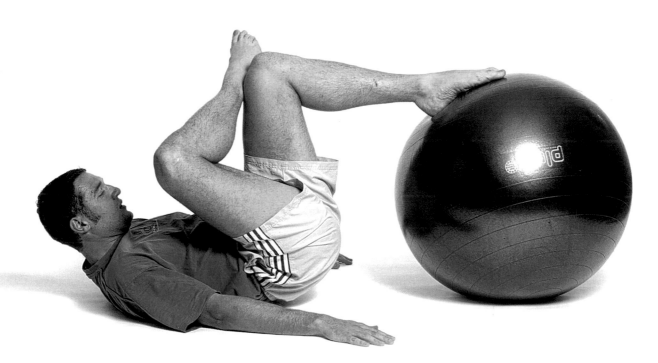

Pull the ball in toward your buttocks until you feel a stretch.

Gluteals Stretch

Level: All

The muscles of the buttock (gluteals) are not only for sitting on, but perform important movements of the hip.

Tight gluteal muscles can result in an imbalance, often causing lower backache and restricted hip movement.

Sit on the ball with feet shoulder width apart. Bring one foot up to rest across the knee of the other leg.

Pull in the stomach muscles and flexing from the hip, bend slightly forward until you can feel a pull in the buttock muscle of the raised leg.

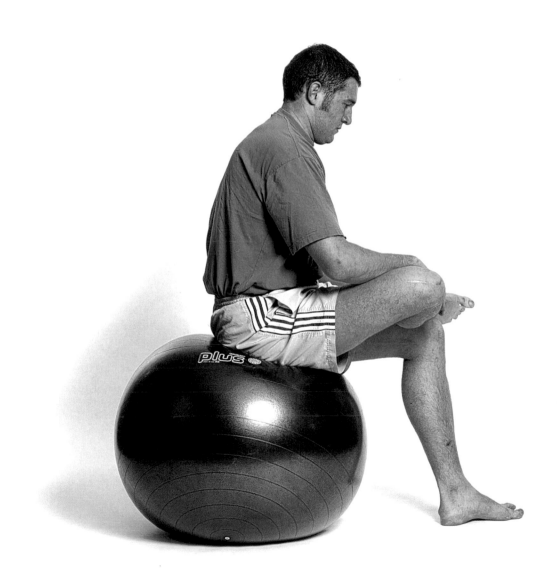

Keep your spine straight as you bend forward.

Hip Flexor Stretch

Level: All

The hip flexor muscles allow us to lift our upper leg from the floor, but they also perform an important stabilizing function for the pelvis and lower back, helping us to maintain balance, posture, and supporting the lower spine.

Stand with the ball slightly to your right side. Lower your weight onto the ball so that it is resting under your right thigh. Pull your spine up straight, gently pushing your pelvis into the ball (not arching your back) until you fell a stretch at the top of the thigh. Hold for 10–15 seconds and release. Repeat three or four times and change around to repeat, using the other leg.

Pull your spine up straight, gently pushing your pelvis into the ball.

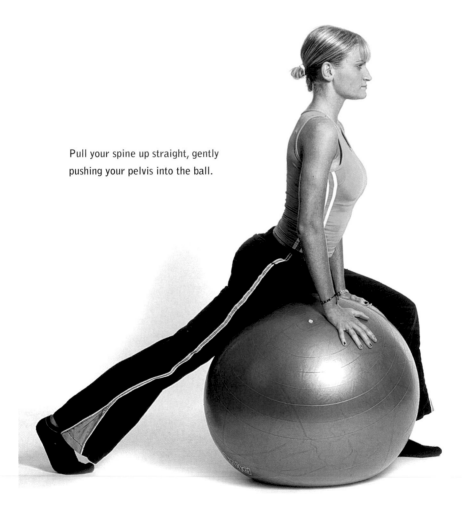

Hamstring Stretch

Level: All

Tight muscles in the back of the thigh (hamstrings) can not only result in injury during sport, but more importantly cause an imbalance pulling on the muscles of the lower back, resulting in poor posture and backache.

Sit on the ball with your legs outstretched in front, shoulder width apart. Tighten the stomach muscles and pull the spine up straight.

Flexing from the hip, slowly reach forward until you feel a stretch in the back of your thigh.

Hold for 10–15 seconds and release. Repeat three or four times.

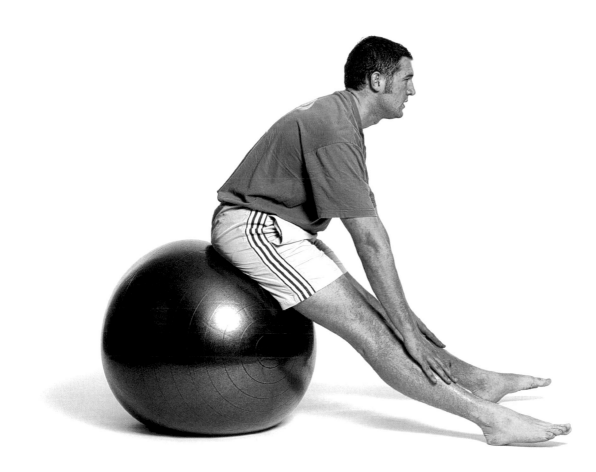

Flex forward from the hips until you feel a stretch behind your thigh.

Adductor Stretch

Level: All

If the muscles on the inside of the thigh (adductors) are too tight, they can become strained (groin strain) during sport or exercise.

Sit on the ball with your feet shoulder width apart.

Keeping your spine straight, stretch one leg out to the side until you can feel a pull on the inside of the thigh.

Hold for 10–15 seconds, relax, and repeat three or four times. Repeat using the opposite leg.

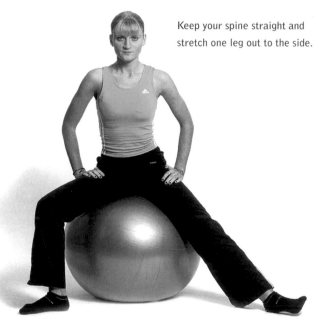

Keep your spine straight and stretch one leg out to the side.

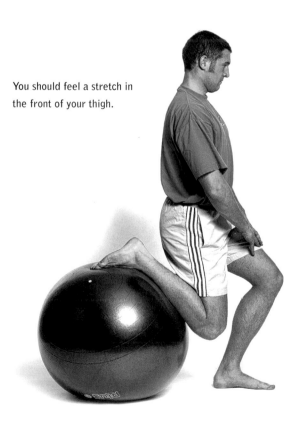

You should feel a stretch in the front of your thigh.

Quad Stretch

Level: All

The muscles in the front of the thigh (quadriceps) are one of the most powerful muscle groups in the body and as such are prone to tightening after exercise, especially after sports that involve running or kicking.

Stand with the ball slightly behind you.

Place one leg so that your shin is resting on the ball. Keeping a straight spine, bend the other leg until you can feel a stretch in the front of the thigh on the ball.

Hold for 10–15 seconds, release and repeat three or four times. Repeat using the other leg.

Pectoral Stretch

Level: All

Muscles in the front of the chest (pectorals) move the arm inward across the body.

Any excess tightness in this muscle group can result in postural imbalances (rounded shoulders) and difficulty in being able to move your arm backward.

Kneel on the floor with one hand outstretched on the ball. Gently lower your upper torso toward the ground until you feel a stretch in the front of the shoulder and chest. Hold for 10–15 seconds and release. Repeat three or four times. Do the exercise again using the other arm.

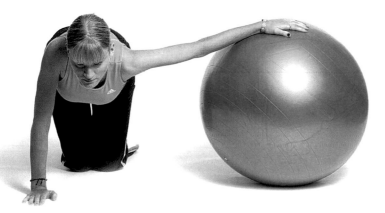

Keep your spine straight as you stretch.

Rotator Cuff Stretch

Level: All

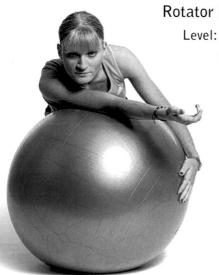

Muscles at the back of the shoulder are just as important as those at the front. An imbalance in these muscles can result in poor movement and pain when performing even the simplest of everyday tasks such as putting on jackets and brushing your hair.

Kneel on the floor or exercise mat with the ball in front of you at chest level.

Place one arm on the ball so that the palm is facing up. Slowly push the ball across your body to the opposite side, until you feel a stretch in the back of the shoulder.

Hold for 10–15 seconds, relax and repeat three or four times. Repeat using the other arm.

Gently push your arm across to the opposite side.

Core Stability

What is core stability?

The lower spine is inherently unstable in its own right. It has to rely on surrounding muscle groups (the core) for support, much the same way as the guy ropes holding up a tent post.

The muscles which form the "core" are the smaller spinal muscles and those of the trunk and pelvic girdle. In short, everything between the ribs and hips.

Core stability is all about training the body to use these muscle groups while carrying out any activity. When the core muscles are functioning correctly, movements become more precise and stable which results in:

- Improved posture and breathing
- Increased muscle strength
- Improved speed and agility
- Reduced risk of injury

Back pain sufferers often find that training the core muscles, at even a basic level, can greatly improve their condition.

Before commencing this section, ensure that you are able to perform the exercises in the "Neutral Alignment" section correctly. This should not be rushed and can take anything from an hour to a few weeks to perfect.

Beginners' Exercises

Basic Bridge

Level: Basic

The bridge is used as a start position in many exercises and it is important that you can master this basic technique in order to train the core muscles safely and effectively.

If this exercise is carried out correctly, the gluteal, hamstrings, pelvic stabilizers, lower back, and abdominal muscles are used in order to maintain stability.

Lay on the exercise mat with your arms in a relaxed position by your side, place your feet on the ball so that the ball is just resting under the lower legs.

Raise the pelvis from the floor by tightening the buttock muscles so that the body is diagonal from shoulders to feet.

Remember to maintain neutral spine alignment and do not allow the back to arch.

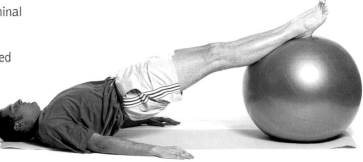

Bridge with Leg Lifts

Level: Basic

Raising one leg from the ball alternately encourages strength in the muscles at the back of the thigh and buttocks (hamstrings and gluteals), while training balance and control in the stabilizing muscle groups.

Lay on the exercise mat with your arms in a relaxed position by your side, place your feet on the ball so that the ball is just resting under your lower legs.

Using the gluteal and hamstring muscles, raise the pelvis from the floor so that your body is diagonal from shoulders to feet. Slowly raise one leg from the ball and hold for a few seconds. Return and repeat using the other leg. The ball must stay as still as possible.

Remember to maintain neutral spine alignment and do not allow your back to arch.

Start with the basic bridge position.

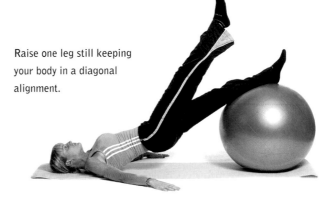

Raise one leg still keeping your body in a diagonal alignment.

Bridge and Double Knee Flex

Level: Basic

The action of pulling in the ball with the feet strengthens the hamstring and gluteal muscles. The aim of this exercise is to control the motion of the ball so that movement is smooth. The ball should not wobble and your spine should not be allowed to drop toward the floor.

Lay on the exercise mat with your arms in a relaxed position by your side. Place your feet on the ball so that the ball is just resting under the lower legs.

Using the gluteal and hamstring muscles, raise your pelvis from the floor so that your body is diagonal from shoulders to feet. Holding this position, use your feet to pull the ball in toward your buttocks. Slowly return to the straight leg position, still keeping your pelvis off the floor. Remember to maintain neutral spine alignment and do not allow your back to arch.

Flex your knees and, controlling the ball with your feet, pull it in toward your buttocks.

Start with the basic bridge position.

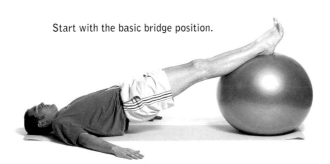

Reverse Bridge

Level: Basic

The reverse bridge forms the basis of many of the exercises in this book and needs to be executed correctly in order to achieve the best results and avoid injury. Lay with the ball under your shoulders and your feet flat on the floor shoulder width apart.

Flex your knees at a 90 degree angle.

Tighten the stomach muscles and maintain neutral alignment.

Hold this position for as long as you can and practice this until it becomes easy.

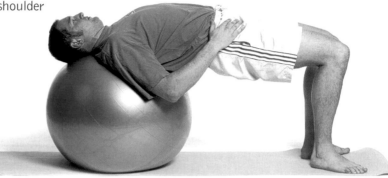

Basic reverse bridge position.

Side Walk

Level: Basic

Walking sideways with the ball trains the core and deep abdominal muscles to maintain neutral posture and alignment while moving.

Lay with the ball between your shoulders in the reverse bridge position and your feet shoulder width apart. Tighten your lower abdominal muscles.

Hold your arms out horizontally to either side and slowly walk sideways so that the ball rolls from one shoulder to the other.

Keep the knees, hips, and shoulders in line and do not allow the back to sag or arch during movement.

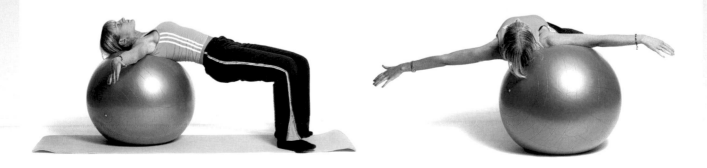

Start with the reverse bridge position.   The ball needs to pass from one shoulder to another.

Hip and Knee Flexion

Level: Basic

The core muscles are further challenged during this exercise as the body attempts to maintain stability while flexing each leg at the hip alternately.

Control has been mastered when this exercise can be performed without the ball moving or the spine sagging or arching.

Lay with ball under your shoulders and your feet shoulder width apart.

Tighten the lower abdominal muscles and flex one leg at the hip to 90 degrees.

Hold for a few seconds, then return your leg to the floor and repeat using the other leg.

Do not allow the back to arch or sag during this exercise.

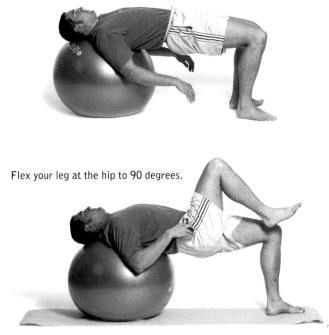

Start with the reverse bridge position.

Flex your leg at the hip to 90 degrees.

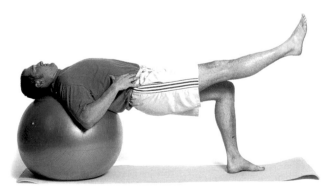

Lift one leg from the floor keeping it straight.

Reverse Bridge with Leg Extension

Level: Basic

Again, the aim of this exercise is to strengthen the core muscles and improve balance (proprioception).

The brain and muscles learn to maintain alignment and stability, while each leg is lifted and held from the floor.

Lay with the ball under your shoulders and your feet shoulder width apart.

Tighten the lower abdominal muscles and lift one leg away from the floor, keeping the leg straight.

Hold for a few seconds, then return your leg to the floor and repeat using the other leg.

Do not allow your back to sag or arch during this exercise and the ball should be kept as still as possible.

Adductors

Level: Basic

Squeezing the thighs against the ball recruits and strengthens the inner thigh muscles (adductors). Weakness in this muscle group often results in "groin strain" injuries when the body is asked to turn or change direction quickly with the load on one leg.

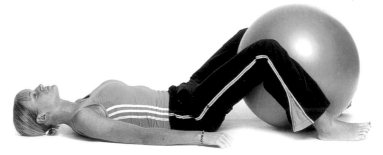

Keep your spine in neutral while squeezing your thighs together.

Performing this simple exercise with the lower abdominal muscles tightened also works the pelvic stabilizers, which need to function in harmony with the adductors.

Lay on the exercise mat with the ball placed between your knees and your arms relaxed by your side.

Tighten your stomach muscles and, keeping your spine and feet firmly on the floor, squeeze the thighs together and hold for a few seconds.

Release and repeat until the muscles begin to fatigue.

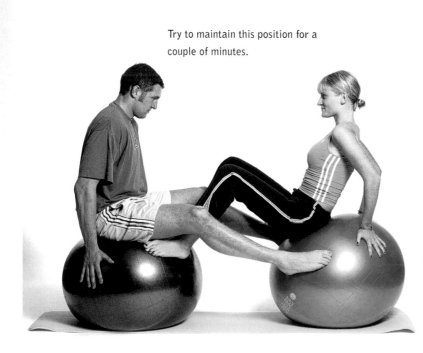

Try to maintain this position for a couple of minutes.

Seated Balancing with Partner

Level: Basic

More fun than an exercise, but not to be taken lightly. Most of the core muscles are recruited as the body tries to gain and maintain balance.

Both partners sit facing each other in a neutral sitting position.

Using one foot at a time, lift each foot and place it on your partner's exercise ball.

Once both partners have achieved balance, try to maintain this position for a couple of minutes until the exercise balls can be held steady quite easily.

Kneeling

Level: Basic

Kneeling on the ball requires strength and coordination from the shoulder and upper leg muscles, as well as the core stabilizing muscles.

You will have to be persistent as this initially takes a lot of practice.

Start by placing your hands and knees on the ball shoulder width apart.

Slowly roll the ball lightly forward to lift your feet from the floor.

You may need a partner to steady the ball or place it against a chair or immovable object until you gain control fully.

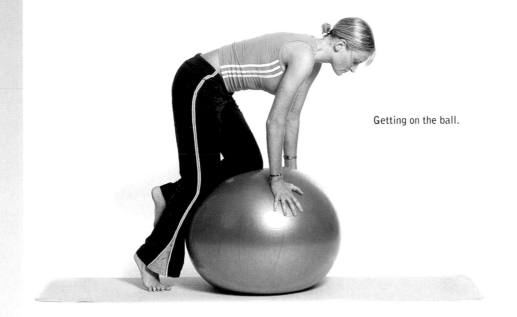

Getting on the ball.

Kneeling position.

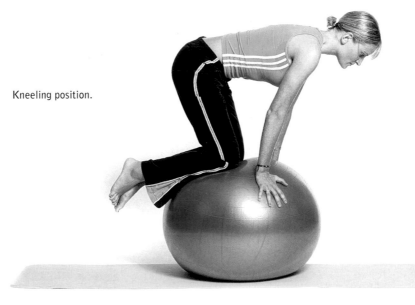

Intermediate Exercises

Bridge with Single Knee Flex

Level: Intermediate

Flexing the hip and knee while maintaining stability of the ball strengthens the hamstrings and the core muscles.

It is important to keep your body in diagonal alignment and not allow your spine to sag or arch.

Lay with your arms in a relaxed position by your side, place your feet on the ball so that the ball is just resting under the lower legs. Using the gluteal and hamstring muscles, raise your pelvis from the floor so that your body is diagonal from shoulders to feet. Flex one leg 90 degrees at the hip and knee, hold this position for a few seconds, and return to the start position. Repeat with the other leg.

Learn to extend the length of time you can hold this position. Move the arms in toward the body to make the exercise harder.

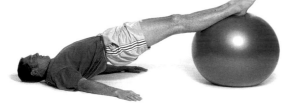

Start with the basic bridge position.

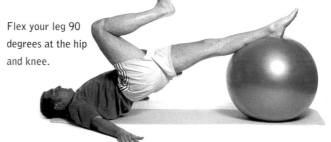

Flex your leg 90 degrees at the hip and knee.

Bridge with Leg Weights

Level: Intermediate

Adding ankle weights to this exercise means that you are now lifting the legs against resistance making the hamstring, gluteal, and core muscles work harder.

Wearing ankle weights, lay on the exercise mat with your arms in a relaxed position by your side. Place your feet on the ball so that the ball is just resting under your lower legs.

Using the gluteal and hamstring muscles, raise your pelvis from the floor so that your body is diagonal from shoulders to feet. Slowly raise one leg from the ball and hold for a few seconds. Return and repeat using the other leg. The ball must stay as still as possible.

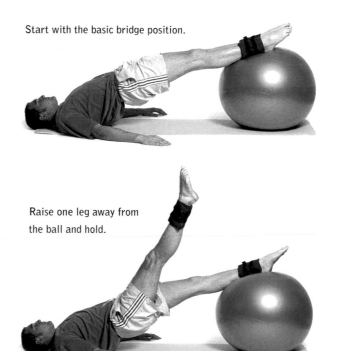

Start with the basic bridge position.

Raise one leg away from the ball and hold.

Reverse Bridge and Leg Extension with Band

Level: Intermediate

Introducing the resistance band into this exercise recruits the quadriceps of the leg as it is raised while the hamstring, gluteal, and core muscles work to keep the body in neutral and the ball stable.

Put a knot in the resistance band so that it is slightly taut when it is placed around your feet, shoulder width apart. Place the resistance band under your right foot and around your left ankle. Lay with the ball under your shoulders in the reverse bridge position.

Tighten the lower abdominal muscles and lift one leg away from the floor pulling the resistance band until your leg is straight. Hold for a few seconds, then return your leg to the floor, and repeat using the other leg.

Do not allow the back to sag or arch during this exercise.

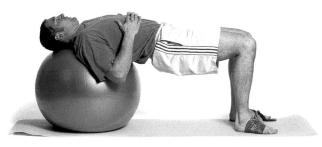

Start with the reverse bridge position and a resistance band around both feet.

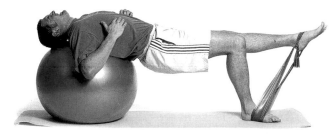

Lift one leg until extended fully.

High Bridge

Level: Intermediate

This is a harder version of the bridge position using the feet on the ball instead of the lower legs. Calf muscles in the lower leg are exercised as well as the hamstring, gluteal, and core muscles.

While maintaining the diagonal alignment from shoulder to knee, it is important not to place any stress on the neck.

Lie on the exercise mat with your feet planted flat on top of the ball, with your arms placed by your sides. Tighten your lower abdominal muscles.

Slowly raise your pelvis from the floor keeping your knees flexed and feet on the ball until your body is diagonal from feet to shoulders. Hold for a few seconds and slowly return to the start position and repeat.

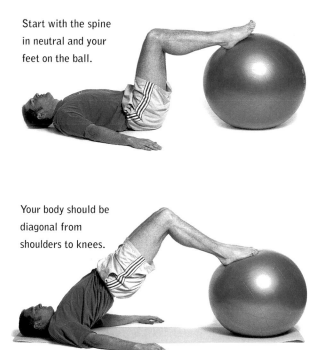

Start with the spine in neutral and your feet on the ball.

Your body should be diagonal from shoulders to knees.

Reverse Bridge with Cushion

Level: Intermediate

Placing the stability cushion under the feet makes balancing more difficult, requiring more strength from the hamstring, gluteal, and core muscle groups.

The brain now has to learn to balance the foot at the same time as the shoulders.

Lie with the ball under your shoulders and your feet shoulder width apart placed on a stability cushion.

Tighten the lower abdominal muscles and lift one leg away from the floor, keeping the leg straight.

Hold for a few seconds, then return the leg to the floor and repeat using the other leg.

Do not allow your back to sag or arch during this exercise. Keep the ball as still as possible while limiting the wobbling of the foot on the cushion.

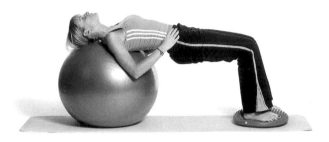

Start with the spine in neutral.

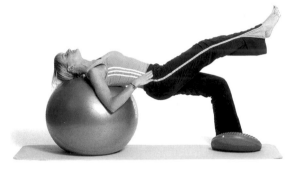

Raise one leg away from the floor.

Leg Circles

Level: Intermediate

The aim is to learn to control the leg from the hip joint, working the deep rotators of the leg to improve the range of movement, strength, and stability from the hip joint.

This is a simple action, but is often performed incorrectly causing damage in the knee and ankle joints. It is important to turn out from the hip and keep the knee and ankle joints firmly fixed, imagining your leg is "splinted."

Lay on the exercise mat with your feet on the ball and your arms relaxed by your side.

Tighten the lower abdominal muscles and raise the right leg from the ball about 45 degrees, slowly turn the leg outward from the hip and, keeping the knee and toes fixed in line, draw circles in the air making sure the movement comes from the hip.

Draw a few small circles until the leg begins to fatigue.

Return the leg to the ball and repeat with the left leg.

The spine must stay in neutral with no hollow between your back and the floor.

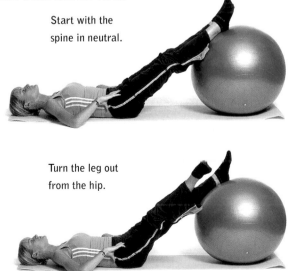

Start with the spine in neutral.

Turn the leg out from the hip.

Sitting Balance

Level: Intermediate

Simply practicing sitting on the ball and lifting your feet from the floor is an ideal way to train the core stabilizing muscles.

Adding weight into the equation changes your center of gravity, making it harder to lift your feet from the ball and maintain stability.

Sit on the ball with your spine in neutral and feet shoulder width apart. Hold your arms out in front or at either side to aid stability.

Leaning slightly backward, slowly raise both feet a few inches from the floor. Hold for a few seconds and return to the start position. Try to keep the ball as static as possible. You can progress this exercise further by holding a medicine ball in front of you or crossing your arms over your chest.

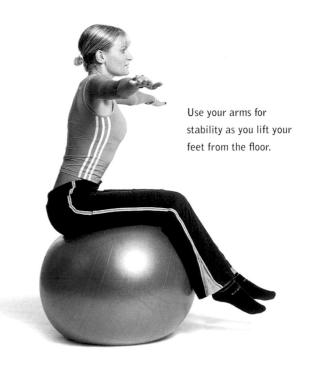

Use your arms for stability as you lift your feet from the floor.

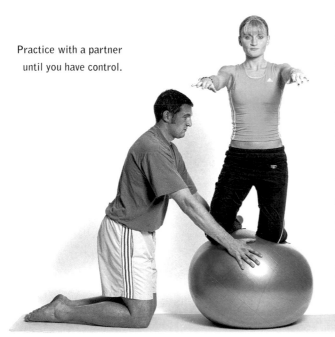

Practice with a partner until you have control.

Intermediate Kneeling

Level: Intermediate

This exercise requires strength from the quadriceps and coordination of the core stabilizers and hamstrings.

Although this position will seem almost impossible to achieve at first, the brain quickly adapts to new situations and practice is the key to success.

Kneel on the ball with your arms outstretched for added stability. The ball should be under your shins and is controlled by using the quadriceps and the feet. Try to get your spine as straight as possible without losing balance.

Practice with a partner holding the ball until you feel you have control.

Advanced Exercises

Advanced Reverse Bridge with Cushion

Level: Advanced

This exercise introduces movement to the top of the body, while maintaining balance in the reverse bridge position.

The aim of this is to keep neutral alignment while performing another task, thus increasing core strength and coordination.

Lay with the ball under your shoulders and your feet shoulder width apart on a stability cushion. Hold a dumbbell out in front of you at chest level.

Tighten your lower abdominal muscles and maintain stability, while at the same time moving the dumbell in an arc from your head to your knees and from one hand to the other.

The upper torso must not move position and the spine must be kept in neutral. The only movement should come from the shoulders and arms.

Do not allow your back to sag or arch during this exercise.

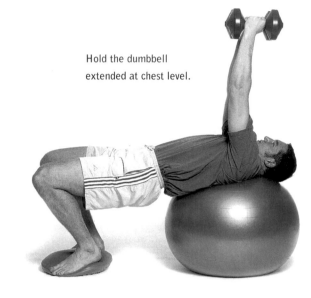

Hold the dumbbell extended at chest level.

Cushion and Ball Bridge

Level: Advanced

By now you should be used to performing the bridge position without difficulty. In order to make the muscles and brain work harder, introduce the stability cushion under the shoulders. The degree of difficulty will depend on how far the cushion is inflated as putting more air in the cushion will decrease stability.

Lie on the exercise mat with a stability cushion under your shoulders and arms in a relaxed position by your side, place your feet on the ball so that the ball is just resting under the lower legs.

Using the gluteal and hamstring muscles, raise your pelvis from the floor so that your body is diagonal from shoulders to feet. Slowly raise one leg from the ball and hold for a few seconds. Return it and repeat using the other leg. The ball must stay as still as possible.

Your body should be diagonal from shoulders to feet.

Cushion Bridge with Leg Weights

Level: Advanced

Wearing ankle weights will strengthen the quadriceps on the leg being lifted as well as producing a new gravitational force for the core muscles to cope with.

Wearing ankle weights, lie on the exercise mat with a stability cushion under your shoulders, your arms in a relaxed position by your side, and your feet on the ball so that it is just resting under your lower legs.

Using your gluteal and hamstring muscles, raise your pelvis from the floor so that your body is diagonal from shoulders to feet. Slowly raise one leg from the ball and hold for a few seconds. Return and repeat using the other leg. The ball must stay as still as possible.

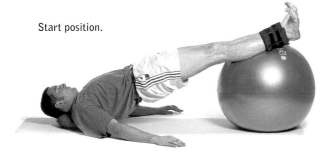
Start position.

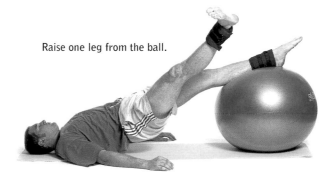
Raise one leg from the ball.

Bridge with Dumbbells

Level: Advanced

By now you should have mastered control of the core muscles in the bridge position. Performing dumbbell presses in this position trains the brain and muscles to maintain stability while performing another function, just as the body will be required to do in work and sporting situations. Using ankle weights and dumbbells gives us the resistance to strengthen the muscle groups involved.

Wearing ankle weights, lie with the cushion under your shoulders, your feet on the ball so that it is just resting

under the lower legs, and hold dumbbells in each hand with palms facing inward.

Using the gluteal and hamstring muscles, raise your pelvis from the floor so that your body is diagonal from shoulders to feet.

Bring the dumbbells out in front of you at chest level, keeping the ball as still as possible.

Return and repeat using the other leg.

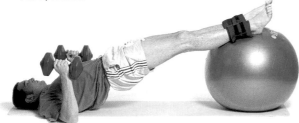
Start position.

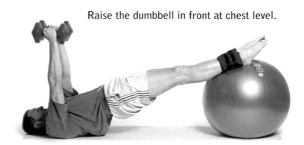
Raise the dumbbell in front at chest level.

Cushion Bridge with Dumbbells

Level: Advanced

The bridge and dumbbell exercise is advanced by adding a stability cushion between the shoulders and the floor. This creates more instability, which in turn makes the brain and muscles work harder in order to maintain balance. Moving the upper and lower limbs simultaneously will improve coordination.

Wearing ankle weights, lie on the exercise mat with a stability cushion under your shoulders. Place your feet on the ball so that it is just resting under your lower legs. Hold dumbbells in each hand, palms facing inward. Using the gluteal and hamstring muscles, raise your pelvis from the floor so that your body is diagonal from shoulders to feet. Slowly raise one leg from the ball and hold for a few seconds. At the same time bring the dumbbells in front of you at chest level. Return and repeat using the other leg. The ball must stay as still as possible.

Reverse Bridge with Medicine Ball

Level: Advanced

Having to work both the upper and lower limbs from an unstable base in this position, strengthens the hamstring, gluteal, and core muscles, while making the brain work even harder to maintain stability and improve coordination.

Lay with the ball under your shoulders and feet shoulder width apart placed on a stability cushion. Hold the medicine ball at chest level.

Tighten the lower abdominal muscles and lift one leg away from the cushion keeping the leg straight. At the same time extend the medicine ball out in front, keeping it at chest level. Hold for a few seconds, return your leg to the floor, and the ball to a resting position. Repeat using the other leg.

Do not allow the back to sag or arch during this exercise.

Start position.

Hold the medicine ball at chest level.

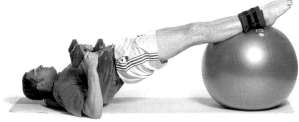

Press the dumbbells out at chest level and raise your leg from the ball.

Extend the medicine ball and lift one leg from the cushion.

Hip and Knee Flexion with Cushion

Level: Advanced

This position maintains stability of the ball and neutral alignment while performing a controlled movement in the lower limbs. Coordination, strength, and balance are improved.

Lie with the ball under your shoulders and your feet shoulder width apart on a stability cushion.

Cross your arms over your chest. Slowly flex your right leg at the hip to bring your knee toward your chest while the other leg stays on the cushion. Hold for a few seconds and return to the start position. Repeat using the other leg.

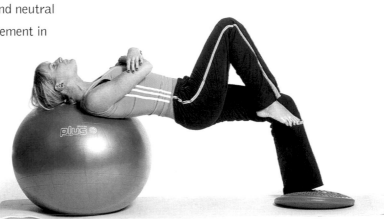

Slowly flex your leg at the hip and bring your knee toward your chest.

Advanced Hip and Knee Flexion

Level: Advanced

Ankle weights are added to make lifting the lower limbs more difficult and forcing the brain and muscles to work much harder in order to achieve stability.

Wearing ankle weights, lay with the ball under your shoulders and feet shoulder width apart on a stability cushion.

Hold the medicine ball at chest level. Slowly flex the right leg at the hip to bring your knee toward your chest, while lifting the medicine ball away from your body. Hold for a few seconds and return to the start position. Repeat using the other leg. Maintain the stability of the ball and a neutral alignment.

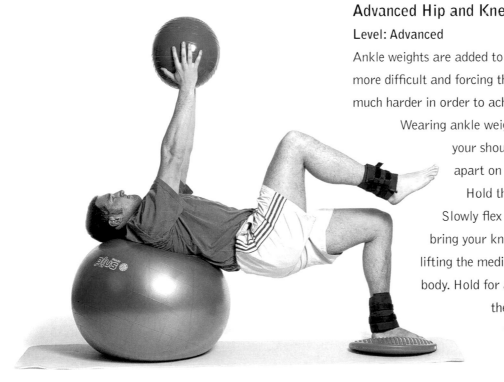

Lift the medicine ball away from your body as you raise your leg from the ground.

35

Leg Circles with Weights

Level: Advanced

Again, the emphasis here is on turning out the leg from the hip and not the knee or ankle joint.

Adding weights makes it harder to control the leg, building strength in the adductor and pelvic stabilizing muscles.

Wearing ankle weights, lie on the exercise mat with your feet on the ball and your arms relaxed by your side.

Tighten the lower abdominal muscles and raise your right leg from the ball about 45 degrees, slowly turn the leg outward from the hip and draw circles in the air a few times.

Return the leg to the ball and repeat with the left leg.

Remember to turn out from the hip.

Kneeling with Leg and Arm Extended

Level: Advanced

This one will require the help of a partner until you achieve control. Once you are able to do this alone, you can consider your core stability to be in excellent shape, as nearly every muscle group in the body will be working either actively or in a stabilizing role to keep you on the ball.

Adopt the basic kneeling position with your hands and knees on the ball.

When you have achieved balance, slowly extend the left leg behind and the right arm out in front. Try to maintain a neutral spine position throughout. When you can do this easily, try changing to the opposite arm and leg.

Raising one arm and leg tests core stability in this position.

Group Kneeling

Level: Advanced

Once you have mastered the upright kneeling technique, try doing this as a group. It is an ideal way to practice throwing and coordination skills in a team environment.

Adopt the intermediate kneeling position and working with a partner or in a group practice sports specific skills, such as throwing a ball to each other.

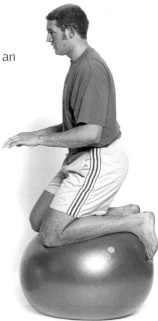

Upright kneeling position.

Double Ball Sitting

Level: Advanced

This may look easy, but the body is having to control two moving objects at the same time, so it is a real test of balance and coordination skill.

Actually getting your feet onto the second ball is the hardest part of the exercise.

Sit on one ball, and place one foot on a second ball in front, then slowly lift the other foot and place it on the second ball shoulder width apart, with your knees slightly flexed.

Maintain a neutral spine and practice sitting in this position. Once mastered, try using light upper body weights.

You can get a partner to assist or wedge the second ball against a wall until you feel safe enough to do this on your own.

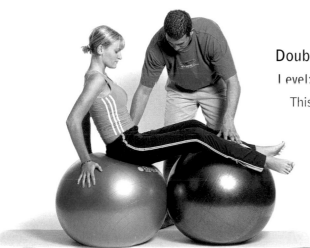

Ask a partner to help get your feet onto the second ball.

Maintain a neutral spine.

Abdominals

The muscles of the abdomen perform a vital function in supporting the lower spine, protecting the internal organs and helping us breathe as well as allowing us to twist, rotate, and sit up. Weakness or dysfunction in this muscle group can lead to:

- Excess curvature of the lower back
- Protruding, weakened stomach muscles
- Inability to stabilize the pelvis when lifting one leg

Abdominal muscles are large, extending from the ribs to the pubic bone and out to the sides. The four main sections form a natural "corset" crossing over each other in different directions.

Nearly all the exercises in this book will work the abdominal muscles in their stabilizing capacity, but the ones in this section are designed to strengthen and tone the muscle group, improving posture, spinal strength, and lung function.

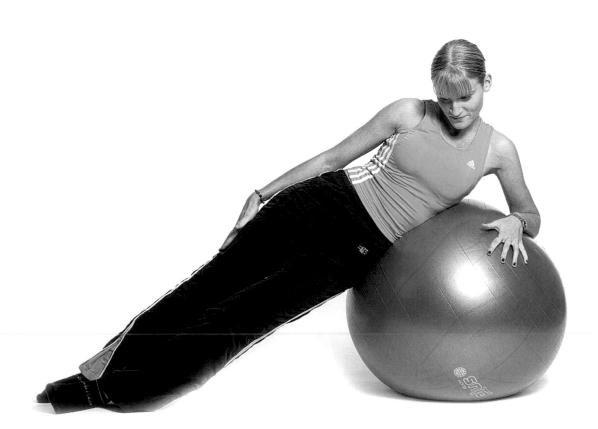

Beginners' Exercises

Lower Abdominals

Level: Basic

The lower abdominal muscles play an important part in the core stabilization of the pelvis, as well as supporting and strengthening the lower spine.

Simply leaning backward on the ball puts these muscles under contraction, strengthening them without risk of injury to the spine.

Sitting on the ball with feet shoulder width apart, lean backward, moving the ball forward with your pelvis. Keep the spine straight as you do this.

When you feel the lower abdominal muscles tighten, hold for five seconds and return to a seated position by pulling in the pelvis.

Repeat until the muscles begin to fatigue. To make the exercise harder, cross your arms over your chest and try holding for longer periods.

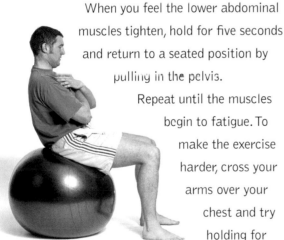

Cross your arms over your chest to make the exercise more difficult.

Use outstretched arms for balance.

Sitting Crunch

Level: Basic

This exercise will work the muscle that gives you the "six pack" appearance (*rectus abdominis*).

Control of this muscle group helps to protect the lower spine and improve posture and breathing.

Lay with the ball under your lower spine and feet placed shoulder width apart. Keeping your feet firmly on the floor, slowly lift your shoulders forward.

Return to the start, repeating the exercise until your stomach muscles begin to fatigue.

Remember to place your hands either side of the head so as not to pull on the neck.

Altering the position of the ball between the pelvis and the shoulders allows you to work the upper, middle, and lower parts of the muscle.

Start with the ball under your lower spine.

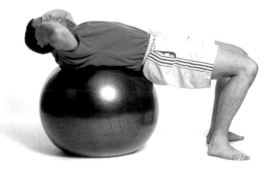

Lift your shoulders from the ball.

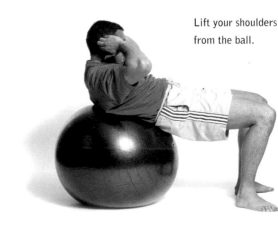

Crunch

Level: Basic

Placing your feet on the ball works the abdominal muscles just a little harder, but at the same time the brain is having to concentrate on balancing the object beneath your feet, which increases the stabilizing ability of the muscles being worked.

Lay on the floor or exercise mat with both heels resting on the ball, your hips and knees at 90 degrees. Tighten the lower abdominal muscles and breathe steadily into the rib cage.

Place hands either side of your head (do not pull on your neck) and lift your shoulders from the floor toward your knees for a few seconds, then release and return to starting position.

Repeat until the lower abdominal muscles begin to fatigue.

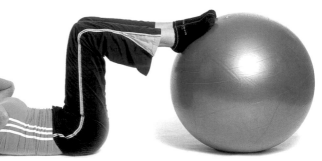

Lift your shoulders from the floor toward your knees.

Side Crunch

Level: Basic

Although this is a basic exercise designed to work the muscles, which bend the spine from one side to another, it is very important for core stability.

Do not be surprised if you have difficulty laying on the ball in this position to start with, until your sense of balance (proprioception) improves.

Lay with the ball under one side and your feet placed against a wall, one in front of the other.

Lay on your side crossing your arms over your chest.

Lift your upper torso from the ball.

Cross your arms over your chest and squeeze your shoulder blades together to prevent rounding.

Slowly raise your upper body from the ball and hold for a few seconds, then return to the start position. Remember to keep the alignment of your knees, hips, and shoulders throughout.

Hip Flexors

Level: Basic

Control of the hip flexors is important in most sports to aid balance and agility. Training these muscles while seated on the ball adds an extra unstable dimension, making the brain work hard to keep the ball still. In order to do this, many muscle groups are used including the smaller, deeper muscles of the spine.

Sit on the ball with your spine in neutral. Tighten the lower abdominals. Lift one leg from the floor by flexing at the hip and then extend the knee to straighten the leg as far as possible. Hold for a few seconds and return to the start position. Repeat with the other leg. Maintain control of the ball and your posture throughout.

Double Leg Lift

Level: Basic

This exercise may seem very difficult at first until core stability improves, but practice is the key here in order to train the brain and muscle groups to act together.

The abdominals, spinal muscles, and gluteals are recruited among others, making this a very effective balance training technique.

Sit on the ball with your spine in the neutral position and feet shoulder width apart. Tighten the lower abdominal muscles. Slowly lift your feet from the floor using your arms to stabilize yourself. Try to hold for a few seconds and release.

Make the exercise harder by crossing your arms over your chest.

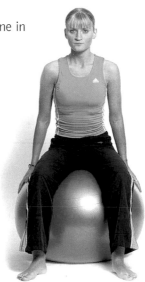

Seated start position.

Flex at the hip.

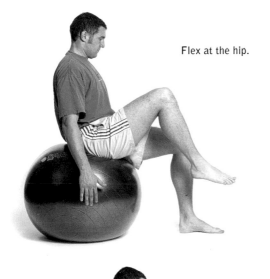

Extend the knee.

Use your arms to aid your balance as you raise your feet from the floor.

Intermediate Exercises

Lower Abdominals

Level: Intermediate

Resistance in the form of a medicine ball, held in front of the body, means that the lower abdominals need to work harder allowing you to progress a simple exercise to its next level.

Sit on the ball and hold a medicine ball (not too heavy) out in front at chest height. Lean backward moving the ball forward with the pelvis.

When you feel the lower abdominal muscles tighten, hold for five seconds and return to a seated position by pulling in the pelvis. Maintain the position of the medicine ball directly in front of your chest throughout the exercise.

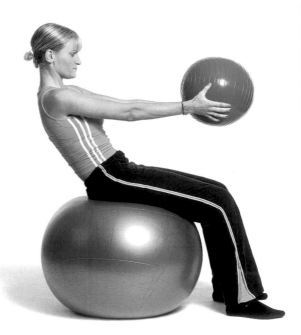

Lean back holding the medicine ball at chest level.

Intermediate Crunch

Level: Intermediate

The action of grasping the ball under the knees already puts the larger abdominal muscle (*rectus abdominis*) into contraction and allows you to isolate and train the area closer to your chest (upper fibers). When the exercise is performed in this position, the "pull" is felt much higher up in the abdomen, under the rib cage.

Lie on the floor or exercise mat. Grasp the ball under your knees and lift from the floor. Tighten the lower abdominal muscles and place your hands either side of your head.

Slowly lift your shoulders from the floor toward your knees, remember not to pull on your neck. Hold for a few seconds and return your upper body to the start position. Repeat until the abdominal muscles begin to fatigue.

Start with the ball held under your knees.

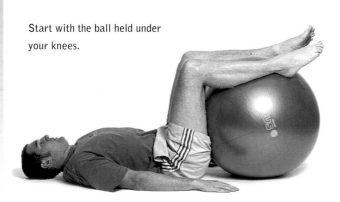

Slowly lift your shoulders toward your knees.

Intermediate Side Crunch

Level: Intermediate

Adding the medicine ball or a dumbbell into this exercise places resistance on the muscle group being worked and, consequently, the muscles are strengthened as they have to work harder to achieve contraction.

The brain also has to cope with the added weight in front of the torso changing the way it has to think about balancing your body on the ball.

Lay with the ball under one side and your feet placed against the wall, one in front of the other with your knees slightly bent. Hold a medicine ball at chest level and squeeze your shoulder blades together to prevent your shoulders from rounding. Slowly raise your upper body from the ball and hold for a few seconds, returning slowly to the start position.

Sitting Obliques

Level: Intermediate

Training the muscles, which run diagonally from the side to the center of the abdomen (obliques) is important for strength and stability. Doing this exercise on an unstable base such as the ball, not only strengthens the muscle group but also activates the stabilizing muscles at the same time.

Sit on the ball and roll forward with the pelvis until it is under the lower spine. Place your hands either side of your head. Raise the upper body toward the knees and over to the left side, at the same time lift the left leg toward the right shoulder. Hold for a few seconds and slowly return to the start position.

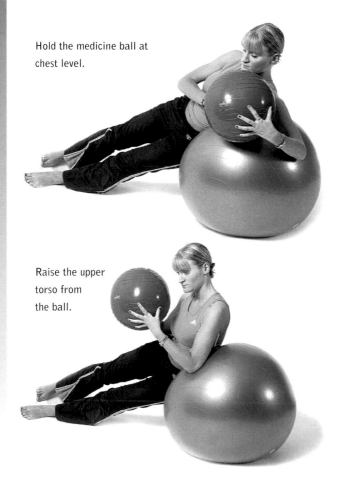

Hold the medicine ball at chest level.

Raise the upper torso from the ball.

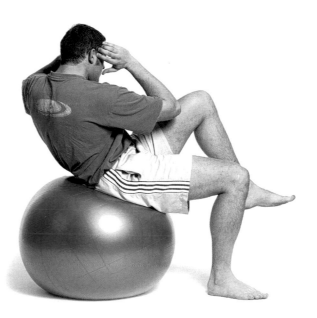

Lift the left leg to the right shoulder.

Obliques

Level: Intermediate

Very different from performing oblique exercises in a seated position, this exercise concentrates on maintaining a neutral spine position while working the muscles which flex, side bend, and rotate the trunk (internal and external obliques). The emphasis here is on the external obliques.

Lie on the floor or exercise mat with the ball under your heels with your hips and knees at 90 degrees

Tighten the lower abdominal muscles. Reach down one side to touch the ball, keeping the body firmly on the floor and taking care not to allow the back to arch. Hold for a few seconds, return to the start position, and repeat on the other side.

Reach down toward the ball keeping the spine in neutral.

Seated Obliques with Dumbbell

Level: Intermediate

Here, the obliques are not only having to rotate the trunk over to the opposite side, but they are having to move the added weight of the dumbbell. This helps to further strengthen and build the muscle fibers.

Sit on the ball and roll forward with the pelvis until it is under the lower spine. Hold the dumbbell firmly with both hands at chest level. Raise the upper body toward the knees and over to the left side, at the same time lift the left leg toward the right shoulder.

Hold for a few seconds and slowly return to the start position. Repeat lifting the right leg and left shoulder.

Raise the upper body toward the knees at the same time lift the left leg toward the right shoulder.

Intermediate Hip Flexors

Level: Intermediate

Adding another unstable object, such as the stability cushion, advances this exercise by making balance much more difficult. The brain has to really start working the stabilizing muscles in order to stop you from falling from the ball.

Sit on the ball with your spine in neutral and feet placed on the stability cushion. Tighten the lower abdominals. Lift one leg from the floor by flexing at the hip and then extend your knee to straighten your leg as far as possible. Hold for a few seconds and return to the start position. Repeat with the other leg. Maintain control of your posture and the ball throughout.

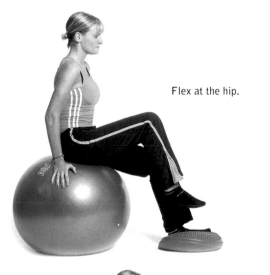

Flex at the hip.

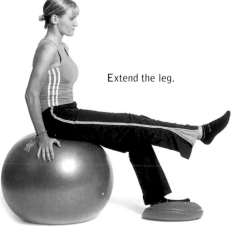

Extend the leg.

Intermediate Double Leg Lift

Level: Intermediate

The ankle weights are being used in this exercise, simply to alter the center of gravity and make the exercise more difficult to achieve.

The muscles and brain have to work harder in order to keep the feet off the floor and the body balanced on the ball. Wearing ankle weights, sit on the ball in a neutral position with feet shoulder width apart. Tighten the lower abdominal muscles. Slowly lift your feet from the floor using your arms to stabilize yourself. Try to hold for a few seconds and release.

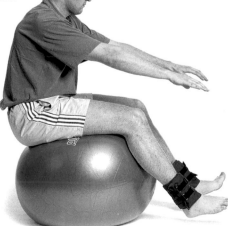

Seated start position.

Use outstretched arms to aid balance.

45

Advanced Exercises

Wall Crunch

Level: Advanced

A highly advanced way to work the *rectus abdominis*. In this position your body has no stability at all and is relying purely on the strength of the stabilizing muscle groups to maintain the position while carrying out this activity.

Sit on the ball facing the wall. Place your feet firmly against the wall, shoulder width apart. The ball should now be under the lower spine and pelvis.

With your hands on either side of your head, tighten the stomach muscles, and slowly lift your shoulders toward the wall. If this exercise is done correctly, your knees and hips should not move from their original position.

Lay on the ball with your feet against wall

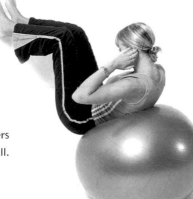

Lift your shoulders toward the wall.

Advanced Crunch

Level: Advanced

By holding the ball between your lower legs and altering the angle at which your legs are held, you will be able to isolate different fibers in the *rectus abdominis* allowing you to work the upper, middle, or lower fibers independently.

Raising the legs higher recruits the upper fibers of the muscle group (closer to the ribs).

Lay on the floor or exercise mat, place the ball between your lower legs. Tighten the lower abdominal muscles and place your hands either side of the head.

Raise your legs 45 degrees from the floor. In this position, slowly lift your shoulders from the floor toward the knees. Hold for a few seconds and lower the upper body back to the floor. Your feet stay at 45 degrees throughout. When this exercise becomes easy, try raising your legs to 90 degrees.

Working the lower abdomen.

Working the upper abdomen.

Advanced Sitting Crunch

Level: Advanced

Adding resistance and instability to a simple seated crunch exercise requires more aggressive control from the stabilizing muscle groups and greater strength from the active *rectus abdominis*.

Sit on the ball with your feet on the stability cushion and knees bent at 90 degrees. Hold the medicine ball or dumbbell at chest level.

Roll backward until the ball is under the lower spine and pelvis. Slowly lift your shoulders forward while maintaining stability of the ball. Hold for a few seconds and slowly return to the start position.

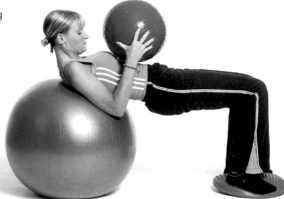

Roll backward until the ball is under your lower back and pelvis.

Advanced Wall Crunch

Level: Advanced

Holding a medicine ball or dumbbell during this exercise gives the resistance required to strengthen the abdominal muscles. The added weight alters the center of gravity, which means the brain and body has to adapt the stabilizing muscle groups accordingly.

Sit on the ball facing the wall. Hold a medicine ball or dumbbell at chest level.

Place the feet firmly against the wall, shoulder width apart, with the knees slightly bent. The ball should now be under the lower spine.

Slowly lift the shoulders toward the wall and hold for a few seconds.

If this exercise is done correctly, the knees and hips should not move from their original position.

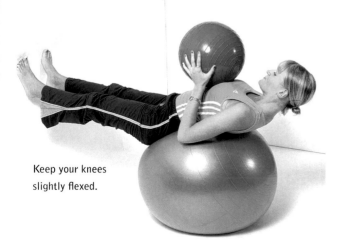

Keep your knees slightly flexed.

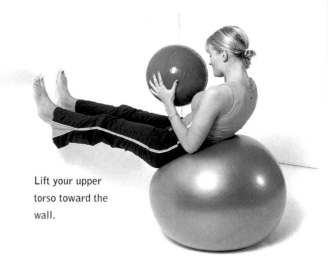

Lift your upper torso toward the wall.

47

Reverse Advanced Abdominals

Level: Advanced

This exercise is for very advanced practitioners only. By lying on the unstable ball and lowering the legs down from a 90 degree start position, you can work the abdominal muscles in reverse, making them contract isometrically (under the body's own weight against gravity). The slower the lowering process, the higher the strain placed on the abdominal muscles, which are now acting as a control muscle group.

Lie with the ball under your lower spine and hands placed against a wall. Tighten your lower abdominal muscles and raise your legs to 90 degrees.

From this position, slowly lower both legs toward the floor as far as you can without losing stability of the ball.

Ask a friend to hold the ball steady until you are sure you have the balance to achieve this alone. Do not let the head hang backward.

Slowly lower your legs toward the floor.

Advanced Side Crunch

Level: Advanced

At this advanced stage you should no longer need the support gained by placing your feet against a wall. Working on the ball in free space now places an added strength dimension to the exercise.

Lie with the ball under one side and your feet on the floor, one in front of the other. Squeeze your shoulder blades together to prevent them from rounding.

Slowly raise your upper body from the ball and hold for a few seconds, returning slowly to the start position.

Your hips and legs should remain static throughout the exercise.

You can then progress this further by crossing your arms over your chest or adding the medicine ball as in the basic and intermediate versions.

Advanced side crunch.

Advanced Obliques

Level: Advanced

Working the obliques in this manner with the body completely destabilized has a twofold function. The muscle group is not only being recruited to lift and rotate the torso, but is also having to act in its stabilizing capacity at the same time.

Sit on the ball with your feet placed on a stability cushion, roll the ball forward with your pelvis until the ball is under the lower spine. Hold the dumbbell firmly at chest level. Raise your upper body toward your knees and over to the right side, and at the same time lift your right leg toward your left shoulder. Hold for a few seconds and slowly return to the start position. repeat using the opposite leg and shoulder. Ask a partner to hold the ball until you are sure you have control.

Ask a friend to steady the ball until you have control.

Advanced Hip Flexors

Level: Advanced

In this exercise, not only is there a completely unstable base from which to work, but adding the ankle weights changes the center of gravity making the muscles and brain work harder to maintain balance and posture.

With ankle weights attached to both legs, sit on the ball with your spine in the neutral position and place both feet on the stability cushion. Tighten the lower abdominals.

Lift one leg from the floor by flexing at the hip as far as possible without leaning backward. Hold for a few seconds and return to the start position. Repeat with the other leg. Maintain control of your posture throughout.

Lift one leg from the floor, flexing at the hip.

Spinal Mobility

Our spine, the vertebral column, is effectively a stack of building blocks one on top of the other with softer discs in between. Its vital functions are:

- Providing protection for the very delicate spinal cord
- Providing attachments for the muscles that move us in different directions
- Allowing us to walk upright
- Flexibility, enabling us to bend, twist, and flex
- Shock absorption

Shaped like an S curve, the spine also has to take the weight of other parts of the body, such as the head, rib cage, and limbs.

Constant weight loading and poor posture, along with the effects of the aging process, lead to the compression and degeneration of the vertebrae, resulting in:

- Pain
- Increased pressure on the intervertebral discs
- Stiffness
- Weakness
- Dysfunction

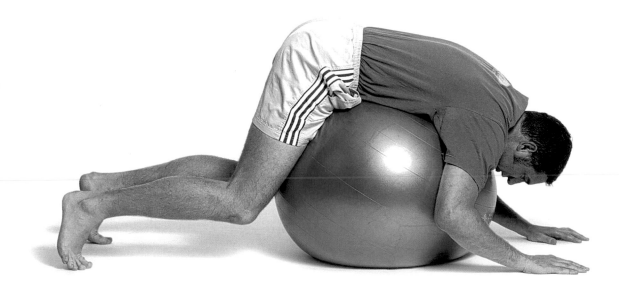

Beginners' Exercises

Pelvic Tilts

Level: Basic

Mobilizing the pelvis from side to side is extremely useful for loosening the lower spine.

Compression in the lumbar vertebrae caused by sitting and degenerative processes, results in lower backache and mechanical dysfunction of the lower spine.

For sportsmen and women, tightness in the lower back can cause a multitude of problems from lack of flexibility to pulled hamstrings and back muscles.

Sit on the ball with your feet shoulder width apart and your arms either side touching the ball.

Tighten the lower abdominal muscles and use the pelvis to push the ball to the left, hold for a few seconds, and return to the start position. Repeat the tilt to the opposite side.

Ensure the spine stays straight and the feet are kept firmly on the floor throughout this exercise.

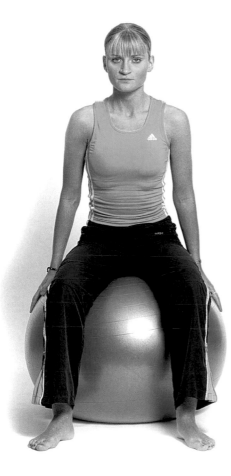

Sit with your feet shoulder width apart.

Keep your spine straight while tilting the pelvis.

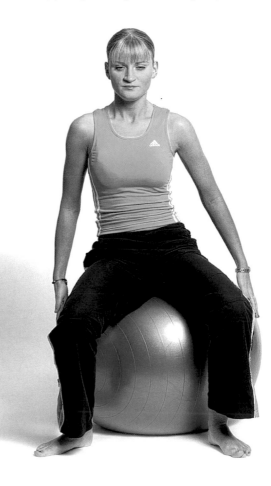

Pelvic Rotation

Level: Basic

Rotating the pelvis while seated on the ball not only loosens the lower spine but also gently works the pelvis and upper leg muscles.

Sit on the ball with your feet shoulder width apart and your hands placed at either side touching the ball.

Tighten the lower abdominal muscles and use the pelvis to slowly rotate the ball in small clockwise and anticlockwise circles.

Ensure the spine is kept straight throughout, if the spine is flexing then try making smaller circles.

Keep your spine straight.

Rotate your pelvis in a circular motion.

Seated Flexion

Level: Basic

This is a similar exercise to stretching sideways over the ball, but this time as you are flexing to one side, the stabilizing muscles on the other side are having to control the movement. A pole is used across the shoulders, merely as an aid to keeping the shoulders level and in a relaxed position.

Sit on the ball with your spine in neutral and your feet placed shoulder width apart, rest the pole across your shoulders and gently grasp it at either side. Keep the shoulders relaxed.

Keeping the pelvis as level as possible, slowly flex the spine to the one side as far as you can, hold for a few seconds, and return to the start position. Repeat to the other side. Do not allow the back to arch or sag during this exercise.

Rest the pole across your shoulders and hold it at either end.

Gently flex to one side keeping your spine neutral and your shoulders relaxed.

Seated Rotation

Level: Basic

The ball supports the lower half of the body in this exercise, while the upper half is rotated to one side then the other. This mobilizes the upper part of the spine (*thoracic vertebrae*) without creating stress on the lumbar spine. The pole is used to keep the shoulders both relaxed and level.

Sit on the ball with your spine in neutral and your feet placed shoulder width apart, rest the pole across your shoulders, and gently grasp it at either side.

Keeping the pelvis level, slowly rotate the spine to the right side as far as you can, hold for a few seconds, and return to the start position. Repeat to the other side.

Do not allow the back to arch during this exercise and always look in the direction you are going.

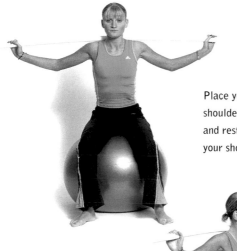

Place your feet shoulder width apart and rest the pole on your shoulders.

Keep your pelvis level as you rotate from one side to the other.

Thoracic Flexion

Level: Basic

This position is often very beneficial to people with back pain. Constant use of the spine leads to compression of the vertebrae, which causes discomfort, pain, and often mechanical dysfunction.

Laying on the ball in this manner, opens up the vertebrae and decompresses the spine while allowing gravity to apply natural traction, easing tension from the spinal muscles.

Kneel on the exercise mat with your upper body over the ball. Keep your eyes looking down so as not to strain the neck.

You should be able to relax in this position, allowing the body to "sag" over the ball.

Stay like this for 30 seconds or more or try rocking gently backward and forward to create relaxing movement in the vertebrae.

Do not hold this position for longer than a minute.

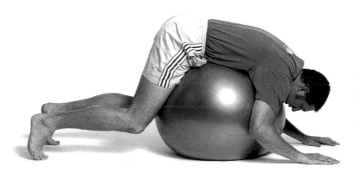

Allow yourself to "sag" over the ball.

53

Extension

Level: Basic

Again, the emphasis is on mobilization of the spine, but this time in extension rather than flexion. Constant sitting, especially with a poor posture, compresses the front of the vertebrae, narrowing the disc spaces, causing pain and dysfunction. Extending over the ball is an ideal way to relax and apply a natural traction to the spine.

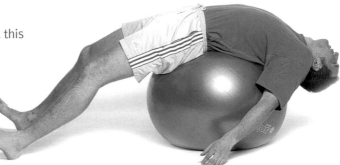

Allow yourself to relax backward onto the ball.

Sit on the ball with your feet shoulder width apart. Slowly roll forward until the ball is under your back. Once in this position, gently allow the spine to extend (arch) backward over the ball. Maintain this position for a few seconds gently rocking back and forth.

Do not allow the neck to extend too far backward. Support your head with your hands, if you feel a strain or if you have neck problems. Get out of this position safely by dropping the pelvis to the floor and rolling off the ball. Do not try to raise torso upward from a flexed position.

Ball Rolling

Level: Basic

This exercise is designed to improve the rotational flexibility of the spine (from side to side).

Movements like this are required in our everyday life and lack of flexibility in this area is a prime cause of back strain in many people.

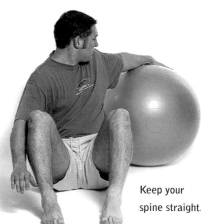

Keep your spine straight.

For sportsmen and women, flexibility in the spine is essential if they are to avoid innocuous muscle strain during activity.

Sit on the floor or exercise mat with your knees slightly flexed, roll the ball around your body from the right around your back to the left.

Maintain a neutral spine alignment throughout and do not rotate further than your body will allow. Flexibility will come gradually with practice. Repeat a few times in either direction.

The shoulder must stay down in a relaxed position and not be allowed to "ride up" while moving the ball.

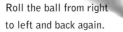

Roll the ball from right to left and back again.

Lumbar Rotation

Level: Basic

This exercise aims to improve lumbar spine mobility. By rotating from side to side on the ball, a rotational force is applied to the vertebrae allowing them to move against each other.

Many people who suffer lower back pain find this exercise invaluable.

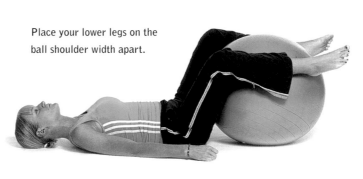

Place your lower legs on the ball shoulder width apart.

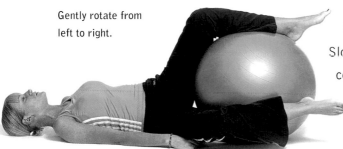

Gently rotate from left to right.

Lie on the exercise mat with your knees flexed, place your lower legs on the ball about shoulder width apart. Gently pull the stomach muscles back to the floor. Slowly rotate the ball from left to right as far as you can comfortably go.

Keep both shoulders firmly on the floor throughout.

Lateral Stretch

Level: Basic

Stretching to one side over the ball, not only mobilizes the vertebrae but stretches the spinal and lateral trunk muscles. The lateral muscles (*latissimus dorsi*) are responsible for controlling arm movements. If these are too tight, shoulder mobility will be impaired.

Kneel on the exercise mat with the ball under the left side. Lift your right arm over your head and push away gently with your outer foot to allow the spine to flex sideways over the ball.

Hold the position for a few seconds and return to the start position. Repeat using the other side. Keep the shoulders, hips, and knees in alignment and do not to allow the spine to arch backward during this exercise.

Keep your alignment as you flex sideways over the ball.

Lumbar Spine Stretch

Level: Basic

During this simple but effective exercise, the ball supports your weight as you flex your upper body forward, letting gravity put a gentle pull on the lower spine.

This also puts a gentle stretch on the hamstring muscles. When the lumbar spine is tight, the hamstrings are usually in the same condition.

Sit on the ball with your feet shoulder width apart and slightly out in front, pull in your navel, and flexing from the hips, hang forward toward your toes.

Keeping the spine straight, maintain this position for a few seconds then return to the start position.

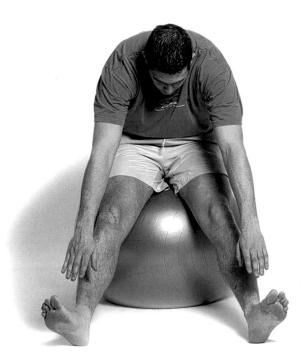

Flex from the hip to hang forward.

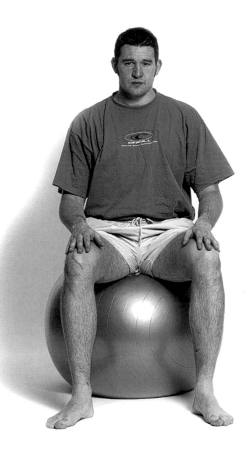

Sit with your feet shoulder width apart.

Intermediate Exercises

Intermediate Pelvic Tilts

Level: Intermediate

Balance and coordination is added to the pelvic tilt exercise by introducing the stability cushion.

Sit on the ball with your feet shoulder width apart, placed on a stability cushion and your arms either side touching the ball or resting on your knees.

Tighten the lower abdominal muscles and use the pelvis to push the ball to the left, hold for a few seconds and return to the start position. Repeat the tilt to the opposite side.

Ensure the spine stays straight throughout by making sure that the back does not hollow or arch.

Intermediate Pelvic Rotation

Level: Intermediate

With your feet on a stability cushion, the leg muscles are having to work harder to maintain balance while the pelvis is being rotated.

Sit on the ball, place your feet on the stability cushion shoulder width apart with your hands at either side, touching the ball or resting on your knees.

Tighten the lower abdominal muscles and use the pelvis to slowly rotate the ball in small clockwise and anticlockwise circles.

Ensure the spine is kept straight throughout, the only movement should come from the pelvis.

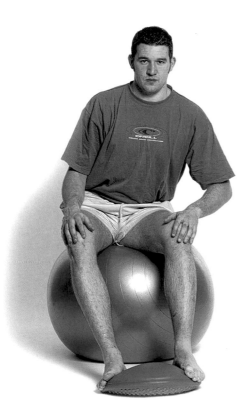

Sit with your feet on a stability cushion.

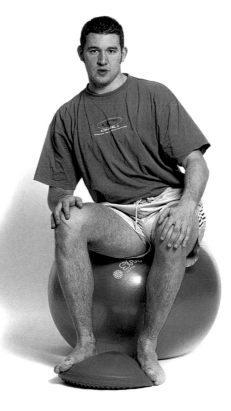

Maintain your balance while rotating the pelvis.

Intermediate Seated Rotation

Level: Intermediate

While rotating the upper torso, the lower half of your body is also having to concentrate on balance.

Sit on the ball with your spine in neutral and your feet placed shoulder width apart on the stability cushion. Rest the pole across your shoulders and gently grasp it at either side. Keeping the pelvis level, slowly rotate the spine to the right side as far as you can, hold for a few seconds, and return to the start position. Repeat the rotation to the other side.

Do not allow the back to arch during this exercise.

Keep the pelvis level as you rotate to the side.

Intermediate Torso Twist

Level: Intermediate

The stability cushion is used as the seat to add an unstable dimension, while passing the ball around the body.

Sit on the stability cushion with your spine in a neutral position and your knees slightly flexed. Roll the ball around your body, passing from your left side around your back to the right. Proceed slowly and only rotate as far as you can comfortably.

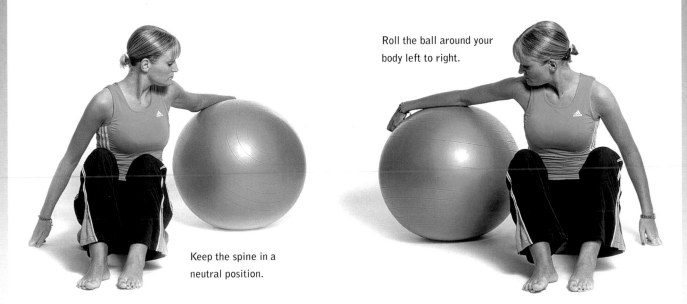

Keep the spine in a neutral position.

Roll the ball around your body left to right.

Intermediate Lumbar Stretch

Level: Intermediate

The stretch in the lumber spine is still the main aim here, but including the stability cushion gives the brain a balance problem to deal with at the same time.

Sit on the ball with your feet shoulder width apart and slightly out in front on the stability cushion, pull in the navel. Flexing from the pelvis, reach forward toward the toes until you feel a slight pull in the muscles at the back of your legs and lower back.

Keeping the spine straight, maintain this position for a few seconds and then return to start position.

Sit with your spine in a neutral position.

Slowly flex forward from the pelvis.

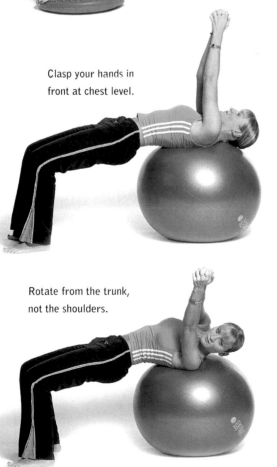

Clasp your hands in front at chest level.

Rotate from the trunk, not the shoulders.

Upper Body Rotation in Reverse Bridge

Level: Intermediate

Designed to activate the trunk rotators, the important thing to remember is that the movement comes from the trunk and not the shoulders.

The hands are held out in front at chest level and are kept in this position throughout to aid in keeping the shoulders level.

Lie with the ball under your shoulders and neck with your feet placed shoulder width apart.

Hold your hands out in front at chest level and maintaining neutral alignment, rotate the arms to the right side rotating from the trunk.

Hold for a few seconds and return to the start position, then repeat to the left side.

Your feet should remain firmly on the floor and your knees should not be allowed to move too far from a central alignment.

Upper Body Rotation with Medicine Ball

Level: Intermediate

Although this exercise can be used to strengthen the trunk rotators, the light weight provided by the medicine ball creates a gravitational pull on the extending muscle groups, aiding in the stretching process. The medicine ball should be relatively lightweight as we are trying to create flexibility and not strength at this point.

Lie with the ball under your shoulders and neck with your feet shoulder width apart.

Hold the medicine ball out in front at chest level and maintaining neutral alignment, rotate the arms to the left side rotating at the waist.

Remember that all movement should come from the torso and not your shoulders.

Hold for a few seconds and return to the start position then repeat to the other side.

Hold the medicine ball in front at chest level.

Keeping a neutral alignment, rotate from the torso.

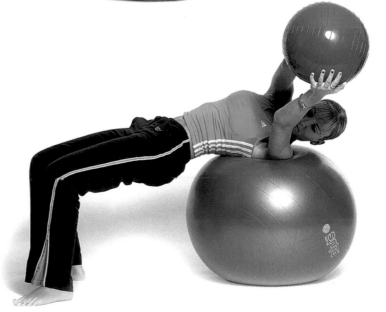

Intermediate Side Flexion

Level: Intermediate

While flexing the spine to the side, the stability cushion is employed to make the brain concentrate on balance at the same time.

Sit on the ball with your spine in neutral and your feet placed shoulder width apart on a stability cushion. Rest the pole across your shoulders and gently grasp it at either side.

Keeping the pelvis level, slowly flex the spine to the right side as far as you can, hold for a few seconds and return to the start position. Repeat to the other side.

Do not allow the back to arch or hollow during this exercise.

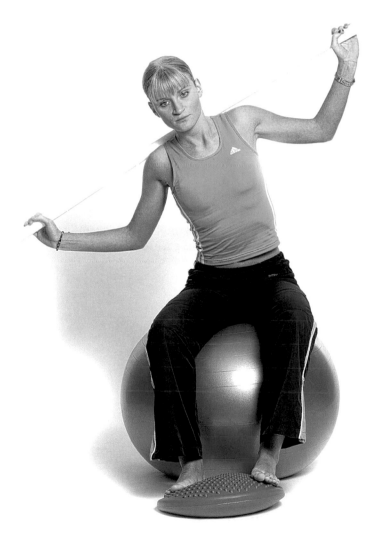

Keep your pelvis level while flexing to the side.

Plank

Level: Basic

The core muscles and the muscles in the back are employed during this exercise, with the aim of building strength and control. Keeping neutral alignment is important if this exercise is to be effective. Kneel on the exercise mat with the ball in front. Place your forearms on the ball and ensure your spine is in a neutral position.

Tighten the lower abdominal muscles and slowly push forward with your feet allowing the ball to roll away from your body, keeping your arms flexed at the elbows. Maintain control of the ball and alignment of the spine throughout.

Hold for about five seconds and slowly return to the start position.

Do not allow the spine to sag or arch throughout this exercise.

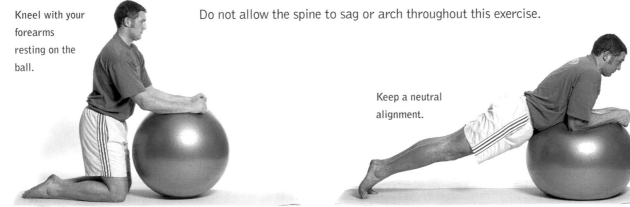

Kneel with your forearms resting on the ball.

Keep a neutral alignment.

Back Extension

Level: Basic

Targeting the larger spinal muscles (*erector spinae*) and the gluteals, this exercise will soon strengthen the muscles of the back.

Kneel on the exercise mat and place the ball under your abdomen and pelvis, feet shoulder width apart.

Holding your arms at either side of your head, slowly raise your upper torso from the ball as far as you can.

Hold for two seconds and slowly lower back to the start position. Keep your back and neck as straight as possible, do not arch the spine or bend the neck.

You can make this exercise harder by bringing the feet closer together.

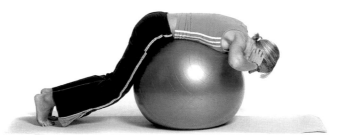

With the ball under your abdomen and pelvis, hold your hands at either side of your head.

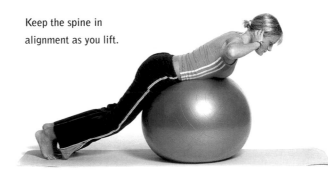

Keep the spine in alignment as you lift.

Trunk Extension and Rotation

Level: Basic

As well as working the large spinal muscles and the gluteals, in this exercise you are also recruiting the deeper intrinsic muscles of the spine, which allow you to extend backward and rotate.

In this instance, we start by using a wall to balance the feet against for stability.

Lay with the ball under your abdomen and with your feet placed against a wall or immovable object.

Place your hands either side of your head.

Slowly lift your upper torso from the ball, rotating toward the center of the spine. Keep your spine and head in alignment throughout. Hold for a few seconds and slowly lower to the start position.

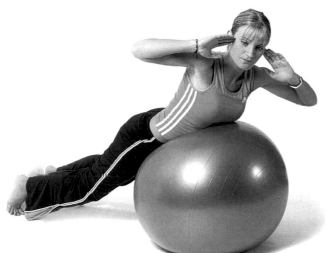

Extend and rotate your trunk from the ball.

Spine Extension

Level: Basic

The object of this exercise is to elongate and stretch the spine. By using the ball as a pivot point it is easier and safer than extending the spine while lying on the floor.

Lie with the ball under your pelvis and stomach. Place your hands on the ball shoulder width apart.

Tighten the lower abdominal muscles and slowly push your pelvis into the ball as you look up and extend your spine away from the ball.

Try to keep a smooth curve from head to toe rather than an arch. Hold for a few seconds and return to the start position. Do not extend your neck backward but keep your head looking forward during this exercise.

Use the pelvis to push into the ball.

Neck Strengthening

Level: Basic

Not only does this exercise help sports people, such as rugby players and racing drivers, but it is highly effective for general everyday use.

Most of us spend great periods of our time with our heads bent forward during our working day. This causes an imbalance in the neck muscles, leading to neck and shoulder pain and even headaches.

Stand with your feet shoulder width apart. Place the ball between the back of your head and the wall.

Ensure a straight posture and using only the muscles of the neck, push your head straight back toward the wall. Your chin should not tip forward and you should remain looking ahead.

Hold for a few seconds and release. Increase this time to make the exercise more difficult

This exercise can be repeated both sideways and forward ensuring that your body is kept in good postural alignment throughout. Imagine a straight line running down your side passing through your ears, shoulders, hips, and knees.

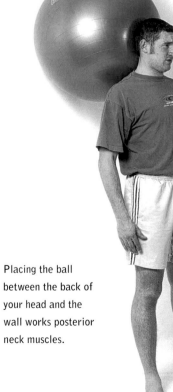

Placing the ball between the back of your head and the wall works posterior neck muscles.

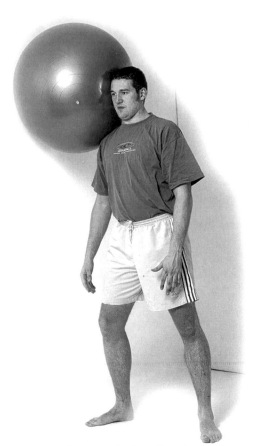

Repeat the exercise from the side.

Intermediate Exercises

Intermediate Plank

Level: Intermediate

This will not only strengthen the muscles of the back but will also work those of the abdomen, legs, shoulders, and arms.

Kneel on the exercise mat with the ball in front. Place your forearms on the ball and ensure your spine is in a neutral position. Tighten the lower abdominal muscles and pushing off with the feet, slowly lean forward, allowing the ball to roll away from the body and extending your legs and arms until almost straight. Maintain control of the ball and the alignment of your spine throughout and do not allow your elbows to lock.

Roll the ball away straightening your arms and legs.

Hold for about five seconds and slowly return to the start position. Do not allow the spine to sag or arch during this exercise.

Plank with Cushion

Level: Intermediate

Adding a stability cushion makes the muscles work harder and further activates the stabilizing muscles, increasing your sense of balance and proprioception.

Kneel with your feet on the cushion and with the ball in front. Place your forearms on the ball and ensure your spine is in neutral. Tighten the lower abdominal muscles and pushing off with your feet, slowly lean forward allowing the ball to roll away from the body and

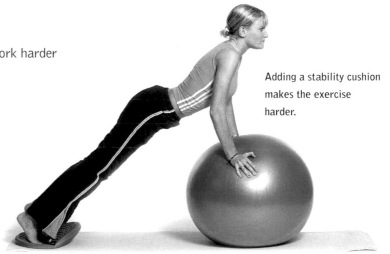

Adding a stability cushion makes the exercise harder.

extending the legs and arms until almost straight. Maintain control of the ball and alignment of the spine throughout and do not allow your elbows to lock. Hold for about five seconds and slowly return to the start position. Do not allow the spine to sag or arch during this exercise.

Plank with Leg Raises

Level: Intermediate

Lifting one leg from the floor changes the center of gravity. The muscles on the weight bearing side are now responsible for holding and balancing the whole body.

Kneel on the floor or exercise mat with your elbows flexed and resting on the ball. The spine should be aligned diagonally from your knees to your shoulders.

Slowly raise one leg from the floor without allowing the spine to arch or sag. Hold for a few seconds and lower to the start position. Repeat using the other leg.

Maintain a neutral alignment.

Intermediate Roll and Return

Level: Intermediate

As the knees are the pivot in this exercise, adding the stability cushion creates a balance problem for the body to deal with. Proprioception and stabilizing muscle strength is enhanced.

Kneeling on the cushion with your hands on the ball, tighten the abdominal and gluteal muscles. You should feel your abdominal muscles begin to work as you roll the ball away from you.

Pivot from the knees allowing the feet to lift from the floor. You should not feel a strain in the lower back during this exercise, tuck your pelvis in further and check your technique if you are experiencing problems.

Keep your spine as straight as possible and do not allow it to arch or hollow in the middle. Maintaining a neutral spine, hold the extended position for about two seconds and slowly return to the start position.

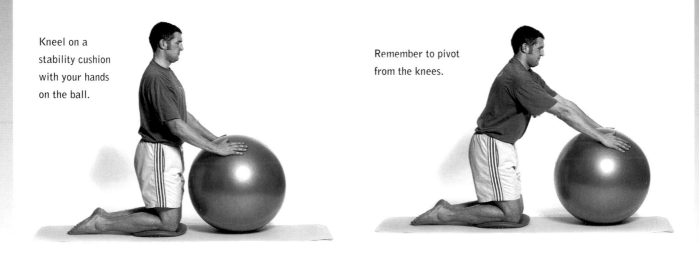

Kneel on a stability cushion with your hands on the ball.

Remember to pivot from the knees.

Intermediate Upper Spine Extensions

Level: Intermediate

Simply adding a medicine ball to the spine extension exercise gives the body added weight. This strengthens and builds the muscles of the spine and trunk.

Kneel on the exercise mat with the ball under your abdomen. Holding the medicine ball at chest level, slowly raise the upper torso from the ball.

If you find you have little room to hold the medicine ball, move further forward placing the ball under the pelvis.

Hold for a few seconds and slowly lower back to the start position.

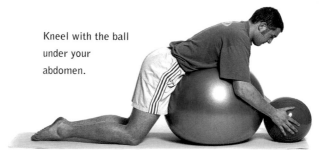

Kneel with the ball under your abdomen.

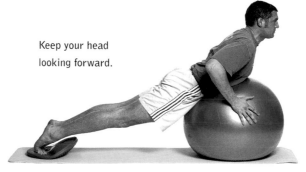

Hold the medicine ball at chest level throughout.

Intermediate Extension

Level: Intermediate

The stability cushion is introduced to destabilize the lower limbs. Spinal extension is coordinated with proprioception and balance.

Lie with the ball under your pelvis and stomach. Place your feet on the stability cushion and your hands on the ball shoulder width apart.

Tighten the lower abdominal muscles and slowly push your pelvis into the ball as you look up and extend your spine away from the ball.

Try to keep a smooth curve from head to toe rather than an arch.

Hold for a few seconds and return to the start position. Do not extend the neck backward but keep your head looking forward during this exercise.

Keep your head looking forward.

Extend away through the spine.

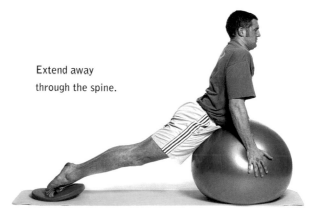

Intermediate Trunk Rotations

Level: Intermediate

Emphasis in this exercise is placed on the trunk rotators, as they are required to move your body and aweight in a particular direction.

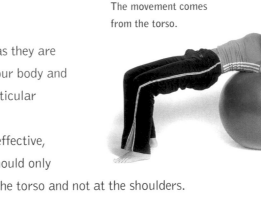

The movement comes from the torso.

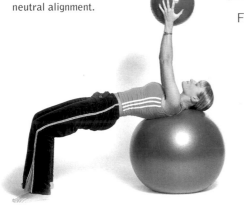

Maintain a neutral alignment.

For this to be effective, movement should only come from the torso and not at the shoulders.

With the ball under your shoulders, tighten the lower abdominals and gently squeeze your knees together by tightening the thigh muscles.

Hold a medicine ball or dumbbell out in front at chest height, rotate the upper torso to the right and hold for a few seconds and return to the start position. Your arms should stay fixed in front of the body throughout.

Repeat to the other side.

Maintain a neutral alignment of the spine with your arms held out at chest level.

Gluteals

Level: Intermediate

The buttock (gluteal) muscles are not just there for us to sit on. All three sets of muscles have important functions and between them, they are responsible for moving the thigh out to the side, turning in and out, and taking the leg backward. An imbalance in these muscles results in uneven stance, poor balance when on one leg, and excess lumbar curvature (sway back).

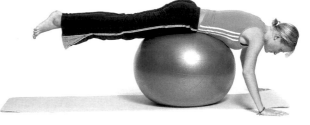

Find a neutral alignment.

Only the gluteals should be working during this exercise.

With the ball under your pelvis and your arms on the floor shoulder width apart, tighten the gluteal muscles to raise the feet upward. Keep the lower abdominal muscles tightened throughout. The ball should be taking most of your weight. Hold for a few seconds and slowly lower back to the start position. Maintenance of this position comes from the contraction of the gluteal muscles.

The lower back must not be allowed to hollow during this exercise.

Allow the ball to take your weight.

Advanced Exercises

Plank with Partner

Level: Advanced

This is an excellent exercise for increasing coordination. The weight of your partner acts as an external force, which your body needs to counteract in order to maintain the position.

Place the two exercise balls in a central position. Rest your forearms on the ball and ensure your spine is in a neutral position. Tighten the lower abdominal muscles and raise your knees from the floor until your legs are almost straight, keeping your arms flexed at the elbows. Maintain control of the ball and alignment of the spine throughout. Hold for about five seconds and slowly return to the start position. Do not allow your spine to sag or arch.

See how long you can hold this position with your partner. Try making things even harder by lifting alternate legs from the floor or try it in groups of three or four.

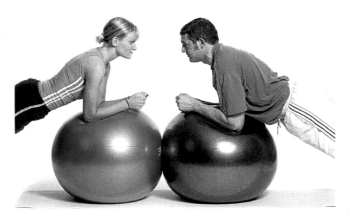

Rest your forearms on the ball and ensure your spine is in neutral.

Advanced Upper Spine Extensions

Level: Advanced

Holding a dumbbell at chest level gives extra weight for the back muscles to lift, which builds and strengthens the muscle groups.

Kneel on the exercise mat with the ball under your pelvis and abdomen. Holding the dumbbell at chest level, push forward with your toes until your legs are almost straight. Slowly raise your upper torso from the ball. Hold for a few seconds and slowly lower back to the start position.

Kneel with the ball under your pelvis and abdomen.

Extend the upper torso from the ball.

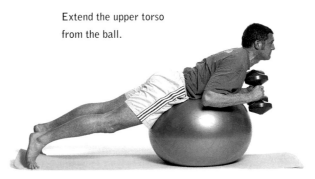

Advanced Plank with Leg Raises

Level: Advanced

Balance is the key aim of this adaptation of the plank exercise. All the weight of the body is being borne by one leg, making the muscles on one side of the spine work much harder.

Kneel on the mat with your elbows flexed and resting on the ball, positioned against a wall. Place your feet on a stability cushion. Push forward with your toes until your legs are straight.

Keeping your spine in a neutral alignment, slowly raise one leg from the floor as far as you can, without letting the lower back hollow.

Hold for a few seconds and lower to the start position. Repeat using the other leg.

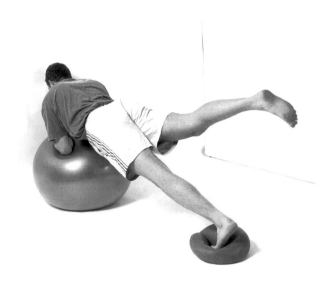

Keep a neutral alignment while raising one leg from the floor.

Standing Roll and Return

Level: Advanced

Rolling the ball in a standing position requires great strength from the abdominal and lower back muscles and should only be attempted if you are very proficient with the roll and return exercises in the kneeling position. The aim is to recreate the stresses required of these muscle groups during sporting or working activity.

Stand with feet shoulder width apart and your hands resting on the ball. Your legs should be flexed at the ankle and knee. The gluteal and the abdominal muscles are pulled in tight.

Roll forward, pivoting from the toes, keeping your hands and arms still and your spine in a neutral position.

Only go as far as you feel safe and ensure your back does not sag or strain too much.

Hold for a few seconds and slowly return to the start position.

If your back is straining, bend your knees further and always keep your head higher than the pelvis. Use a larger ball if you find you are having to reach too far down.

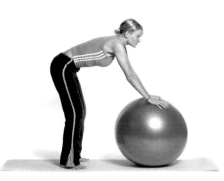

Stand with your feet shoulder width apart, hands resting on the ball.

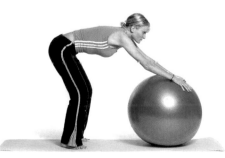

Roll forward, pivoting from the toes.

Advanced Back Extension with Medicine Ball

Level: Advanced

The stability cushion is added to make the body concentrate on balance, as well as strengthening the spinal muscles. Kneel on the cushion with the ball under your pelvis and abdomen.

Holding the medicine ball at chest level, slowly raise your upper torso from the ball.

Hold for a few seconds and slowly lower back to the start position.

Do not allow your head to extend backward or your lower spine to hollow.

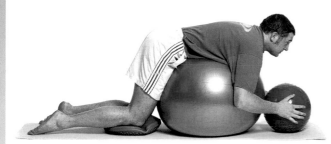

Start with the ball under your pelvis and abdomen.

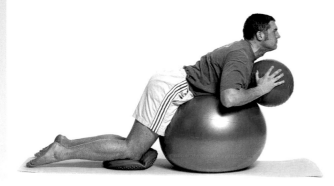

Lift the upper torso from the ball, holding the medicine ball at chest height.

Advanced Trunk Rotations

Level: Advanced

The cushion is used to destabilize the body and make the muscles concentrate on balance as well as strength.

Using the medicine ball adds weight, which will strengthen and build the trunk rotators.

Kneel on the cushion with the ball under your pelvis and abdomen.

Holding the medicine ball at chest level, slowly lift your upper torso from the ball and at the same time lift your right shoulder toward the center of your spine.

Hold for a few seconds and slowly lower to the start position.

Repeat, rotating your left shoulder to the center.

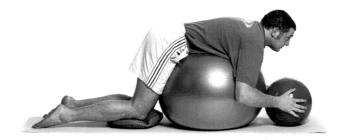

Kneel with the ball under your pelvis and abdomen.

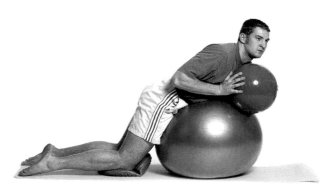

Rotate your right shoulder toward the center of your spine.

Advanced Trunk Rotation with Cushion

Level: Advanced

Use of the stability cushion means that your feet are no longer stable. Now the trunk rotators are working actively to rotate the torso, while the stabilizing muscles in the pelvis and legs are trying to keep the feet balanced.

Lay with the ball under your shoulders and your feet on the stability cushion.

Maintain a neutral spine and hold the dumbbell out at chest level.

Keeping the pelvis still, rotate your upper torso 90 degrees to the right. Hold for a few seconds and slowly return to the start position. Repeat to the other side.

The movement should only be coming from the torso and not the shoulders.

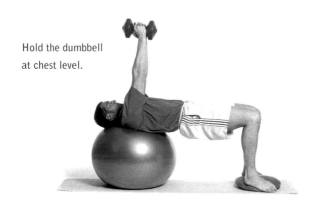

Hold the dumbbell at chest level.

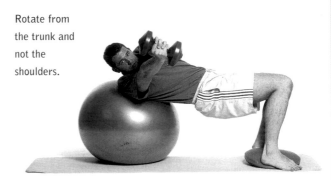

Rotate from the trunk and not the shoulders.

Advanced Glutes

Level: Advanced

This exercise, which is designed to work the buttock (gluteal) muscles, is made harder by adding a stability cushion between the ankles.

The squeezing action needed to keep the cushion between the ankles as the feet are raised, also works the inside of the thigh (adductors). With the ball under your pelvis, place the stability cushion between your ankles. Your arms should be on the floor shoulder width apart.

Tighten the gluteal muscles to raise your feet upward.

Keep the lower abdominal muscles tightened throughout. Hold for a few seconds and slowly lower back to the start position.

Remember that your legs are raised by tightening the gluteal muscles and most of your weight is borne by the ball.

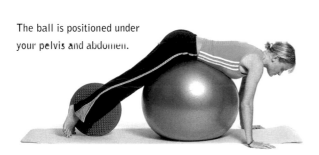

The ball is positioned under your pelvis and abdomen.

Raise your legs upward by tightening the gluteal muscles.

Upper Limbs and Shoulders

The shoulder and arm muscles are recruited in a number of sports and occupations. Racquet sports, swimming, gymnastics, and weightlifting often require the strength and coordination of more than one muscle group.

Each muscle generally has its own particular function, for example to lift the arm forward, upward, or away from the body. In order for the arm to be raised upward and then to perform an overhead serve in tennis, or for a carpenter to drive home a screw into the top hinge of a door, a complex range of synchronized movements has to take place.

Tightness or weakness in these muscle groups can be due to overuse in a particular sport, poor posture, or damage caused by injury. If this imbalance is allowed to continue, the shoulder joint in particular can become unstable, leading to pain, discomfort, limited range of motion, and even disability.

The exercises in this section concentrate on the range of movement in the shoulder and arm joints, as well as improving strength and coordination.

Beginners' Exercises

Shoulder Extension
Level: Basic

This is a basic exercise designed to improve flexibility in the shoulder joint.

Sit on the ball with your feet shoulder width apart. Raise your right arm out in front and lift upward keeping your arm as close to your head as possible. It is important to keep your shoulder down in line with the opposite one, do not allow your shoulder to come up toward the ear.

Start in a relaxed seated position.

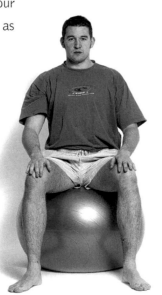

Hold for a few seconds and lower back to the start position. Repeat using your other arm.

Ensure that the lower spine is kept straight and not allowed to arch backward throughout this exercise.

Extend upward as far as you can.

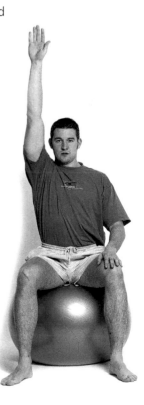

Shoulder Abduction

Level: Basic

Moving and holding your arm out to the side (abduction) is the responsibility of many of the shoulder muscles. Anyone who has an injury to the supporting (rotator cuff) muscles in the shoulder will actually find it difficult to hold the arm in this position.

Sit on the ball with your feet shoulder width apart and your arms by your sides touching the ball.

Lift your right arm straight out to the side as far as you can.

Ensure that your pelvis remains straight and your spine does not arch inward or bend to the side.

Hold for a few seconds and lower to the start position. Repeat using the other arm.

Start in a relaxed seated position.

Keep your spine straight as you extend your arm to the side.

Double Shoulder Extension

Level: Basic

This stretch focuses on the extension of the shoulder joints as the ball is moved up the wall, until your arms are alongside your ears. This also places a mild stretch on the muscles of the chest, which often tighten with tension and everyday activity.

Stand with your feet shoulder width apart facing the wall.

Hold the ball against the wall at chest height.

While keeping the spine straight, roll the ball up the wall as far as you can until your arms are level with your ears.

Hold for a few seconds and lower back to the start position. Do not allow the lower back to hollow during this exercise.

Try to get your arms as high as you comfortably can.

Standing Shoulder Abduction

Level: Basic

The aim of this exercise is to stretch the side (lateral) muscle groups and improve mobility of the shoulder joint.

Stand at 90 degrees to the wall with your feet shoulder width apart.

Hold the ball against the wall at chest height.

While keeping the spine straight, roll the ball up the wall as far as you can without discomfort.

Keep your arm in line with the side of your head. Staying in line with your ear is a good guide.

Hold for a few seconds and lower back to the start position. Repeat using the other side.

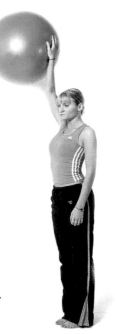

Keep your spine straight and your arm by the side of your head.

Kneeling Shoulder Mobility

Level: Basic

Making sure the shoulder has a full range of movement is just as important in everyday activity as it is in sport.

Keep a neutral spine position.

Using the ball in this position allows you to keep the arm extended, while the ball carries the weight of the limb throughout the movement.

Kneel on the exercise mat with one hand on the ball in front of you.

Keep the spine in a neutral position as you slowly move the ball in an arc from head to toe.

Bring the ball back to the starting position and repeat with the other arm.

Rotate the ball as far as you can.

77

Side Lying External Rotation

Level: Basic

Here the muscles at the back of the joint (*teres minor* and *infraspinatus*) are worked. These muscles are used when the arm is rotated outward or to the side. Weakness in this muscle group often results in pain and restricted use.

Lay with the ball under one side and flex the uppermost arm 90 degrees at the elbow.

Slowly rotate the forearm 90 degrees until your fist is in line with your body. The elbow must be kept firmly fixed by your side. Your shoulder should not be allowed to "ride up." Hold for a few seconds. Repeat using the other arm.

To ensure you are doing this correctly, repeat this exercise while standing and place your hand over the shoulder being worked. You will feel the muscles in the back of the shoulder contract as you move your arm to the side.

Flex your arm 90 degrees at the elbow.

Rotate your flexed arm parallel with your side keeping your elbow firmly in place.

Lateral Stretch

Level: Basic

This exercise stretches the muscles in the side, which attach to the upper arm. If these muscles are tight or injured, simple things like putting on a jacket and brushing your hair can be difficult and painful.

Sit on the ball with your feet shoulder width apart and your spine in a neutral position.

Clasp both arms above your head.

Keeping your spine in a neutral position, gently pull down to the left until you feel a stretch in your right shoulder and under your arm.

Hold for 15 seconds and repeat to the opposite side.

Remember to keep your back from arching during this exercise. The movement should come only from the shoulders.

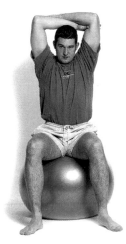

Clasp both arms above your head.

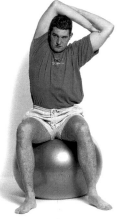

Keep your spine straight as you stretch your arms over to one side.

Chest Press with Ball

Level: Basic

The main muscles at the front of the chest (*pectoralis major*) are responsible for moving the arms inward across the torso. A lack of strength in these muscles reduces the ability to perform inward and downward movements of the arm much like that of the forward crawl in swimming.

The muscles also act as a major stabilizer for the shoulder joint. An imbalance in any of the shoulder muscles results in poor or incorrect movement, often resulting in pain and disability.

Sit on the ball with your feet shoulder width apart. Place a medicine ball at chest height between your forearms flexed at the elbows.

Keeping your shoulders relaxed, gently squeeze your arms together and hold for a few seconds.

The shoulders should not be allowed to move upward or the spine to arch during this exercise.

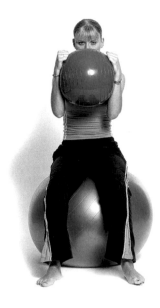

Place the medicine ball between flexed forearms.

Basic Press Ups

Level: Basic

Unlike push ups that are done on the ground, using the ball means that not only are the shoulder and arm muscles being worked, but the muscles of the whole body have to come in to play in order to maintain balance and keep the spine in neutral alignment.

Lie with the ball under your shins and your spine in neutral. Arms at chest height, shoulder width apart.

Keep your head looking forward and do not allow the spine to sag or arch.

Lower your torso using only your arm muscles, hold for a few seconds, and then push back up so that the body is horizontal again. Do not lock your elbows straight. Hold for a few seconds and slowly lower again.

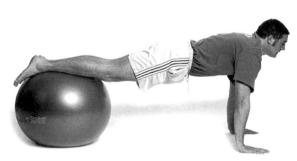

Find a neutral alignment.

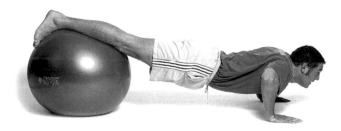

Lower your body to the ground.

Intermediate Exercises

Intermediate Extension

Level: Intermediate

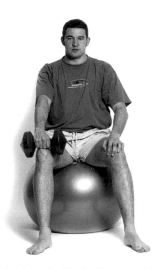

Hold the dumbbell with your palm facing down.

Using the ball as a seat makes it much harder to keep the spine straight while extending the arm.

Lifting the dumbbell out in extension works the teres and deltoid muscles in the shoulder, *latissimus dorsi*, and the triceps.

Sit on the ball with your feet shoulder width apart, holding a dumbbell in one hand with the palm face down.

Raise your arm out in front no higher than 90 degrees (no higher than shoulder height).

Hold for a few seconds and lower back to the start position.

Repeat using the other arm.

Ensure that the lower spine is kept straight and not allowed to arch backward throughout this exercise.

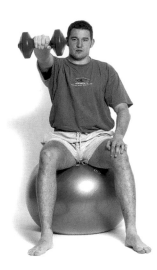

Extend out in front no higher than shoulder height.

Intermediate Abduction

Level: Intermediate

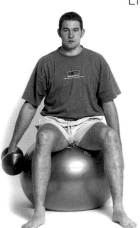

Hold the dumbbell at your side with your palm facing inward.

Lifting the dumbbell out to one side strengthens and builds the deltoid and rotator cuff muscles.

Sit on the ball with your feet shoulder width apart, hold the dumbbell by your side with your palm facing inward.

Lift your arm straight out to the side no higher than 90 degrees (your arm should not come above shoulder level).

Ensure that your pelvis remains straight and your spine does not arch inward or bend to the side.

Hold for a few seconds, then slowly lower to the start position. Repeat using the other arm.

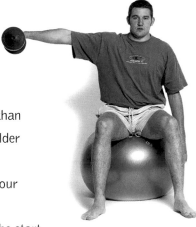

Slowly extend out to the side.

Double Shoulder Extension

Level: Intermediate

This exercise is excellent for loosening the shoulder joint. As the weight of your head and upper body is being suspended by the shoulders, this can also be a very aggressive exercise and should be approached with care.

Lay on the mat with the ball at arms length in front of you. Raise one arm up onto the ball, followed by the other. Keep your head as low to the ground as possible. Hold for a few seconds. Use a smaller ball if you find this exercise too difficult.

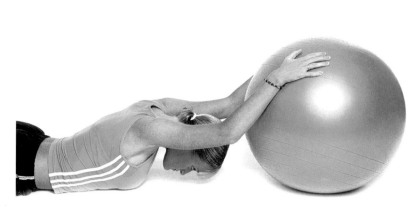

Keep your spine straight as you lower to the floor.

Single Handed Wall Press Ups

Level: Intermediate

The whole weight of the body is borne by the shoulder and arm muscles on one side of the body in this exercise. The stabilizing muscle groups have to work extra hard in order to keep the spine straight.

Stand with your feet shoulder width apart and the ball held firmly against the wall at chest height with one hand. Place the other hand behind your back or by your side.

Keep your spine perfectly straight as you flex the elbow to lower the upper torso toward the ball. Hold for two seconds, then extend the arm back to the start position.

Change hands and repeat with the other side.

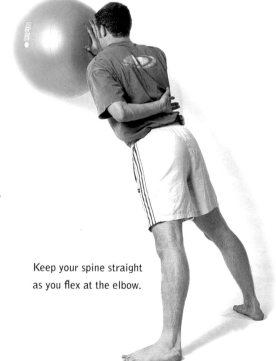

Keep your spine straight as you flex at the elbow.

Bicep Curls

Level: Intermediate

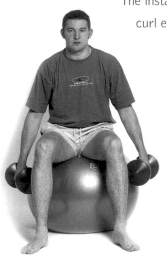

The instability of the ball adds a balance aspect to a simple bicep curl exercise.

Sit on the ball with your feet shoulder width apart. Hold a dumbbell in each hand by your sides with your palms facing inward.

Slowly flex one dumbbell upward, rotating the forearm so that the palm faces the shoulder.

Hold for two seconds and then slowly lower back to the starting position and repeat with the other arm.

It is important not to jerk the movement or hollow the spine in order to lift the dumbbell.

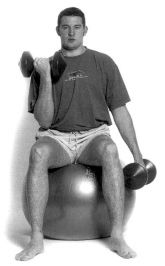

Start with the dumbbells by your side, palms facing inward.

Flex your forearm and rotate so that your palm faces your shoulder.

Triceps

Level: Intermediate

Exercising the triceps is just as important as the opposing muscles group (biceps). The triceps muscles are located at the back of the arm and have three parts (heads). Their function is to extend (straighten) the forearm.

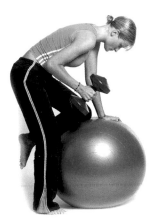

Stand with your left hand and knee firmly on the ball and your right leg slightly flexed so that your torso is parallel with the floor.

Hold a dumbbell in your right hand with your elbow flexed at 90 degrees and your palm facing inward.

Your abdominal muscles should be tightened and your spine in a neutral position.

Keeping your arm close to your side, use only your forearm to slowly move the dumbbell backward until your arm is straight. Hold for two seconds and return to the start position. Repeat using the opposite arm.

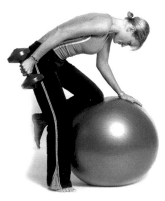

Start with your arm flexed 90 degrees at the elbow.

Extend from your forearm until your arm is straight.

Lateral Pull Downs

Level: Intermediate

The focus in this exercise is on the muscles toward the middle of the back, primarily the *latissimus dorsi* and the lower fibers of the trapezius. Weakness in this area results in poor posture and poor trunk mobility.

Sit on the ball with your feet shoulder width apart on a stability cushion. Tighten the lower abdominal muscles and hold the pole out in front at head height with your arms slightly wider than your shoulders.

Slowly lower the pole down and inward toward your chest. Hold for a few seconds and repeat.

It is important keep your spine straight and your pelvis still.

Incline Bicep Curl

Level: Intermediate

This exercise works the muscles of the upper forearm (biceps), but at the same time makes the body maintain balance against the ball.

The biceps muscles have two parts (heads) and are responsible for flexing (bending) the forearm, turning the palm upward and flexing at the shoulder (moving the arm forward).

Sit on the ball with your arms slightly wider than shoulder width apart and holding a dumbbell in each hand. Roll forward on the ball until it is under the upper torso and shoulders.

Hold a pair of dumbbells by your side, with your palms facing inward.

Slowly flex one dumbbell up toward your shoulder, rotating the forearm so that your palm faces the shoulder.

Hold for two seconds and repeat with your other arm.

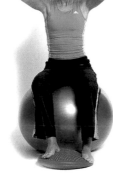

Extend your arms in front at head height.

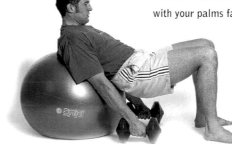

Hold the dumbbells by your sides, with your palms facing inward.

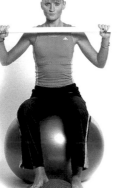

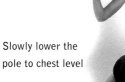

Slowly lower the pole to chest level

Rotate your forearm so that your palm faces your shoulder.

Advanced Exercises

Advanced Wall Press Ups

Level: Advanced

Standing on the stability cushion makes all the stabilizing muscles of the body work all the way down to your ankles, improving proprioception and strength.

Stand with your feet shoulder width apart on a stability cushion and the ball held firmly against the wall at chest height.

Keep your spine perfectly straight as you use your shoulders to perform standing press ups.

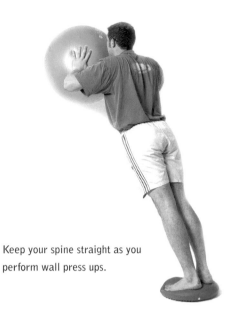

Keep your spine straight as you perform wall press ups.

Push Up

Level: Advanced

Using the stability cushion for the push ups, destabilizes the lower limbs, requiring more balance control from the brain and muscles.

Kneel with your hands on the ball, shoulder width apart and your knees on a stability cushion.

Push the ball away until you can raise your pelvis from the ground creating a diagonal line from head to toes.

Keeping your spine perfectly straight, lift your body away from the ball by using your arm muscles, but do not lock your elbows straight.

Hold for a few seconds and lower until your chest is almost touching the ball again.

Make the exercise harder by moving the cushion and ball further apart.

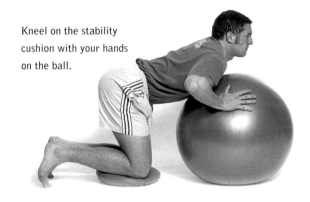

Kneel on the stability cushion with your hands on the ball.

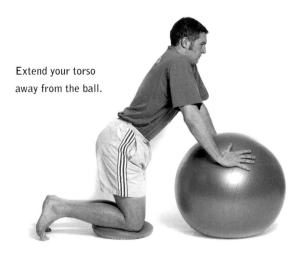

Extend your torso away from the ball.

Advanced Press Ups

Level: Advanced

Lifting one leg from the ball shifts all the body weight onto one side. The stabilizing muscle groups are required to work very hard in order to keep the spine in alignment and the body balanced on the ball.

Lie with only your feet resting on the ball, your spine in a neutral position, and your arms at chest height, shoulder width apart. Keeping your spine in a neutral position, extend one leg from the ball.

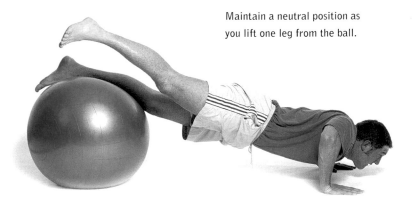

Maintain a neutral position as you lift one leg from the ball.

Lower your torso by flexing at the elbows, hold for a few seconds, and then push back up so that your body is horizontal, but do not lock your elbows straight. Hold for a few seconds and slowly lower again. Repeat, removing the opposite leg from the ball.

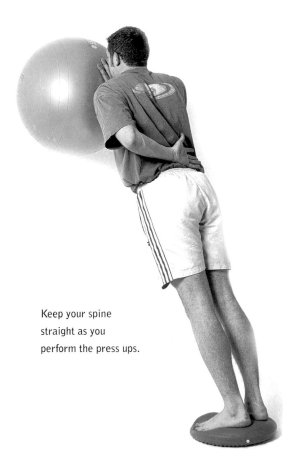

Keep your spine straight as you perform the press ups.

Advanced Single-Handed Press

Level: Advanced

Working single-handed with the ball and standing on the cushion ensures the brain and core stabilizing muscles are working at their maximum to maintain alignment and balance.

Stand with your feet shoulder width apart on a stability cushion. Hold the ball firmly against the wall at chest height with one hand and place the other hand behind your back or by your side.

Keep your spine perfectly straight as you use your shoulder to perform standing press ups.

Advanced Chest Press

Level: Advanced

The stability cushion is placed under your feet to add a challenge to balance and stability.

Lie with the ball under your shoulders and your feet on a stability cushion, adopt the bridge position, keeping the stomach muscles tight.

Hold a dumbbell in each hand with your hands facing inward. Extend your arms outward at shoulder level. Do not let them move backward toward your head.

Slowly lower the dumbbells down as far as you can toward your armpits. Hold for two seconds and then press back to the start position. Do not let your spine sag or arch during this exercise.

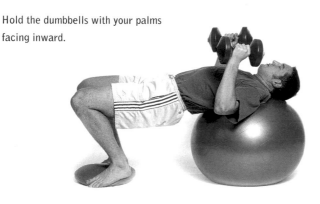

Hold the dumbbells with your palms facing inward.

Extend the dumbbells in front keeping them level with your chest.

Advanced Incline Bicep Curl

Level: Advanced

The stability cushion is added to this exercise, making the quadriceps and hamstrings work to keep the feet stable.

Sit on the ball with your feet shoulder width apart on a stability cushion and holding a dumbbell in each hand. Roll forward on the ball until it is under your upper torso and shoulders.

Extend the dumbbells at either side with your palms facing inward.

Tighten your abdominal muscles and flex the dumbbell up rotating the forearm, so that your palm is facing your shoulder. Hold for two seconds and slowly lower to the start position. Repeat using the other arm.

Do not jerk the movement or arch the back.

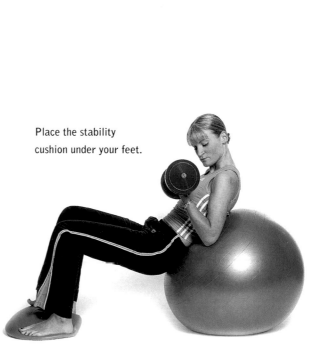

Place the stability cushion under your feet.

Advanced Extension Rotation

Level: Advanced

Strengthen and build the posterior rotator cuff muscles of the shoulder by adding a dumbbell to this exercise.

Laying with the ball under one side, hold the dumbbell with your palm facing inward and your arm flexed 90 degrees at the elbow.

Hold the dumbbell, with your arm flexed 90 degrees at the elbow.

Slowly rotate your forearm away until it is in line with your body, keeping your elbow firmly positioned at your side.

Hold for two seconds and slowly return to the start position.

Place the ball under the opposite side and repeat using the other arm.

Rotate your forearm outward in line with your body.

Advanced Bicep Curl

Level: Advanced

Lengthening a muscle while it is load bearing leads to an eccentric contraction. An eccentric contraction is known to be more effective when using weights to build muscle.

As you are lowering a weight rather than lifting it, you can use a weight 20 to 30 percent heavier than you would use for a bicep curl.

Start with the ball under your torso and roll backward as you lift the dumbbell.

Kneel with the ball under your torso and the arm extended. At the same time as you raise the weight toward your shoulder, roll backward on the ball.

Hold the raised weight for two seconds then roll forward on the ball, gradually allowing your arm to extend back out again and taking at least six seconds to lower the weight.

The longer it takes to lower the weight, the stronger the muscle will become.

Standing Bicep Curl

Level: Advanced

Working the biceps in this position encourages the body to concentrate on balance and alignment. Standing with the ball between your back and the wall, feet shoulder width apart, hold a dumbbell in each hand with your palms facing inward. Tighten the abdominal muscles and keeping the triceps on the ball, flex your lower arm up, rotating your palm toward your shoulder. Hold for two seconds and slowly lower back to the start position. Remember not to jerk the movement or allow your back to arch during this exercise. You can either work each arm independently or both together.

Place the ball between your shoulders and the wall.

Curl the dumbbell up bringing your palm to face your shoulder.

Shoulder Extension

Level: Advanced

Strengthen the shoulder extensors in this exercise by using the ball to aid eccentric contraction. Lowering a weight over a period of time is much more effective at strengthening and building muscles than lifting the weight.

Lay with the ball under your torso and your feet extended shoulder width apart, remaining bent at the knee. Place the other hand on the floor to aid stability.

Start with the ball under your torso.

Holding the dumbbell with your palm facing down, lift the weight until your arm is in line with your head, hold for two seconds and then return your arm back to the starting position, taking at least six seconds to lower the limb completely.

Repeat using the other arm.

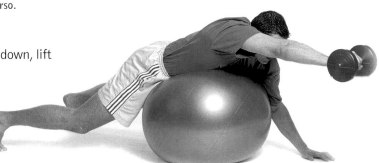

Lift the weight, before slowly lowering it to the start position.

Row

Level: Advanced

This exercise works the *latissimus dorsi*, rhomboids, trapezius, and rotator cuff muscles of the shoulder, along with the posterior fibers of the deltoid and biceps of the arm.

Kneel on the ball with your upper torso almost parallel with the floor. Hold a dumbbell down by your side in one hand with your palm facing inward and balance the other on the ball.

Pull the dumbbell up to touch your rib cage, pulling your elbow back as far as you can and keeping your arm flexed 90 degrees at the elbow.

Hold for two seconds and then slowly lower back to the starting position. Repeat using the other arm.

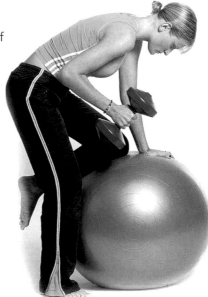

Hold a dumbbell at your side in one hand.

Rotator Cuff

Level: Advanced

This exercise concentrates on the rotator cuff muscles of the shoulder, which are necessary to stabilize the upper arm in the shoulder socket and ensure correct movement of the shoulder joint.

Lie with the ball under your side and your arm resting in front, holding your weight, with your palm facing inward.

Maintaining your stability on the ball and tightening your abdominal muscles, lift your arm out and up so that the dumbbell is now parallel with your body and above your head.

Hold for a few seconds and then slowly lower back to the start position and repeat.

Change sides and repeat using the other arm.

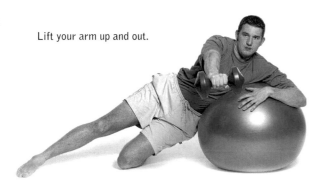

Lift your arm up and out.

Lift your arm out until the dumbbell is parallel with your body and above your head.

Lower Limbs and Pelvis

The muscles of the legs, hips, and buttocks are the focus of this section, with quite an emphasis placed on limb position sense, which is known as proprioception (see page 6).

The leg muscles allow us to flex at the hip, knee, and ankle, enabling us to walk, run, and kick.

The buttock muscles (gluteals) extend the leg backward and out to the side, while also acting as a stabilizing influence during movement.

The hip muscles, in this case the hip flexors, (located at the front of the hip, just above the thigh) play a very important role in stabilizing the pelvis and supporting the lower spine as well as flexing the hip joint.

Strength, coordination, and stability in the lower limb muscle groups are vitally important if we are to walk upright, run, ski, or play soccer.

Nearly all exercises contained in this section will improve the following:

- Strength
- Flexibility
- Stability
- Coordination and proprioception

If limbs are positioned more effectively, especially during sports where changes of direction are needed, then agility and speed should be improved along with a reduced risk of injury, enabling the sportsman or woman to concentrate on his or her skills.

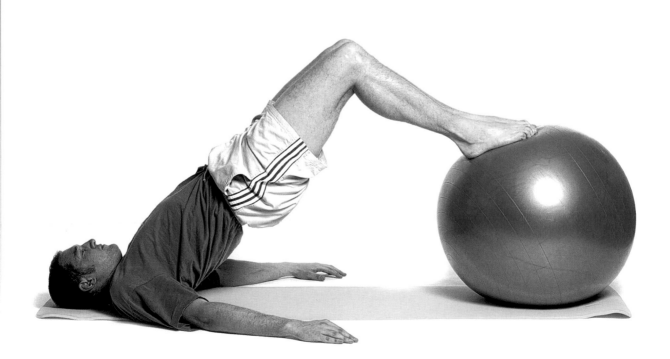

Beginners' Exercises

Toe Touches

Level: Basic

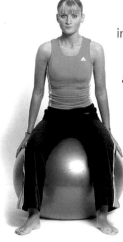

Sit in neutral, your feet shoulder width apart.

Maintaining balance while performing simple movements may seem to be easy. But in these days of spending our lives in cars and office chairs, the smaller intrinsic muscles of the spine can cease to function in the correct way.

Working the lower limbs while seated on the ball encourages mobility and strength in the spine and pelvic stabilizing muscles.

Sit on the ball with your feet shoulder width apart and your hands at either side touching the ball.

Alternately touch each toe on the ground in front of you, keeping the ball as steady as possible.

Remember to start slowly as the object of the exercise is to keep the ball from moving around.

You may find it helpful to hold your arms out in front for balance. When you are confident with your balance, you can speed up the movements.

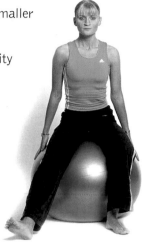

Keep your spine straight as you touch each toe in front.

Marching

Level: Basic

The hip flexors (*psoas* and *iliacus*) more commonly known as the iliospoas, act together to flex the thigh and are the main hip flexor and low back stabilizer. They lie deep in the lumbar spine and pelvis. More often, these muscles are too tight (hypertonic) in most people, resulting in hip and low back problems. The lumbar curve is often exaggerated or reduced.

Sit on the ball with your feet shoulder width apart, hands resting on the ball or holding your arms out in front at chest level to aid balance.

Tighten your lower abdominal muscles and maintain a straight spine.

Alternately, lift each leg from the floor in a marching movement, bringing the knee as high as you can without arching the spine while trying to keep the ball as stationary as possible.

Keep the hip, knee, and toes in line throughout.

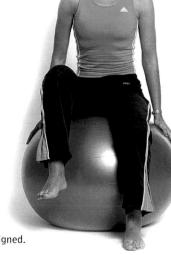

Keep your hips, knees, and toes aligned.

Side Stepping

Level: Basic

Two other muscles, which help to stabilize the pelvis, are the *sartorius* and *gracilis* that lie toward the inside of the thigh. Tension in these muscles can lead to lower back and knee problems.

Sit on the ball with your feet shoulder width apart and your arms held out in front at chest level.

Maintaining a neutral spine, alternately touch your toes out to the side trying to keep the ball steady at the same time.

Start slowly at first as the object of this exercise is to keep the ball as still as possible throughout.

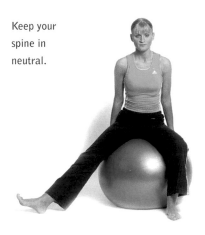

Keep your spine in neutral.

The ball will not move if your balance is controlled.

Hamstrings

Level: Basic

The hamstrings (back of the thigh) are an extremely important muscle group as they have to be a major stabilizing force against the strong opposing group of the quadriceps (front of the thigh). Not only do these muscles need to be flexible, but strength and stability are paramount, especially in sports where the body needs to gain speed and change direction quickly.

Lie with the ball under your head and neck and your arms relaxed or crossed over your chest.

Tighten the lower abdominal muscles and push backward, pivoting from the heel until your legs are outstretched keeping the hips, knees, and toes in line.

You should feel tension in the hamstrings and the gluteal muscles. Hold for a few seconds and return to the start position.

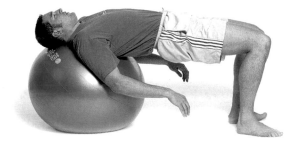

Maintain a neutral spine.

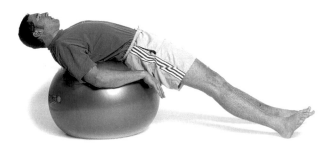

Push back, pivoting from the heels.

Hamstring Curl

Level: Basic

Lie on the floor or exercise mat with your heels on the ball, tighten the lower abdominal muscles. Slowly bring the ball toward the buttocks by tightening the hamstring muscles at the back of the thigh. Control the movement with your feet, so that the hips, knees, and ankles all stay in line. Hold for a few seconds and return to the start position. The spine should not arch away from the floor during this exercise.

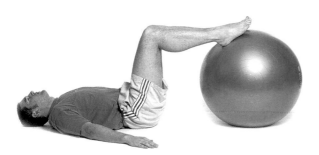

With your spine in a neutral position lie with your feet on the ball.

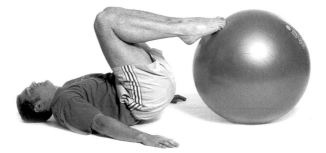

Tighten your hamstrings and bring the ball toward you.

Hamstring Stretch

Level: Basic

A hamstring stretch that also encourages coordination in the lower limbs.

Lie on the floor or exercise mat as close to the wall as possible, place the ball between your feet and the wall. Tighten the lower abdominal muscles. Roll the ball up the wall, keeping it in line with the center of your body, until your knees are fully extended.

Ensure that your spine does not arch from the floor and your stomach muscles remain tight.

Hold for 15 seconds and return the ball to the floor.

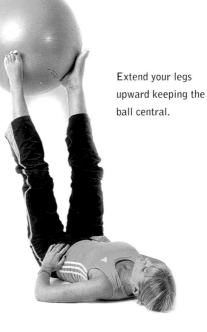

Extend your legs upward keeping the ball central.

Lie as close to the wall as possible.

Single Leg Lifts

Level: Basic

The aim of this exercise is to make the hip flexors and stabilizing muscles work to control the weight and movement of one limb, while also concentrating on balance and alignment.

Sit on the ball with your feet shoulder width apart and arms by your side or crossed over your chest.

Tighten the lower abdominal muscles and slowly lift your right leg from the floor, extending at the knee and keeping it as straight as possible. Hold for a few seconds and return to the start position. Repeat using the other leg. Do not lift the leg higher than your pelvis.

Remember to keep your spine straight, your stomach muscles tight, and the ball as still as possible.

Sit in a neutral position.

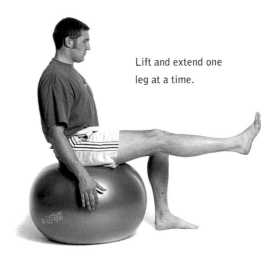

Lift and extend one leg at a time.

Hip Extensions

Level: Basic

Extending your leg out behind your body uses the gluteal muscles to perform the movement and pelvic stabilizers to balance the pelvis and thigh.

Kneel on the floor or exercise mat with the ball under your chest and tighten the lower abdominal muscles.

Slowly extend your left arm and right leg until they are in horizontal alignment with the spine.

Keep your knee and toes pointing toward the floor and in line with your hip.

Hold for a few seconds and return to the start position, repeat using the right arm and left leg.

Do not allow the spine to sag or arch during this exercise.

Extend the opposite leg and arm keeping your spine straight.

Hip Flexion

Level: Basic

The hip flexors (iliospoas) should be controlling this movement, using strength to pull the ball in and stability to keep it in line with the body during movement.

Lie with the ball under your stomach and roll forward until the ball is under your shins. Tighten the lower abdominal muscles and maintain a neutral alignment of the spine.

Slowly bring your knees toward the chest, by pulling in the hip flexors (not bending the spine), ensuring that the lower spine is not allowed to sag or arch.

Hold for two seconds and slowly return the ball to the start position by extending the legs.

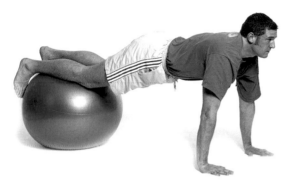

Roll forward until the ball is under your thighs.

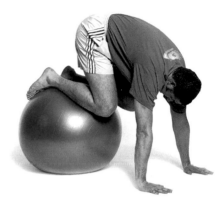

Flex your hips to bring the ball up to your chest.

Lunges

Level: Basic

For the body to be stable in this position requires strength from the quadriceps (front of the thigh) and control from the opposing group (hamstrings).

With the other foot balanced on the ball, even more instability is created as all the body weight is transferred to the leg on the ground.

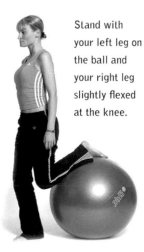

Stand with your left leg on the ball and your right leg slightly flexed at the knee.

Stand with the ball under your left shin and the right slightly bent at the knee.

Maintaining a neutral spine, lunge forward so that the right leg is in a semi-squat position and the left leg is extended on the ball.

Hold for a few seconds then straighten the right leg to return to the start position. Repeat with the other leg.

Do not allow the spine to arch backward during this exercise.

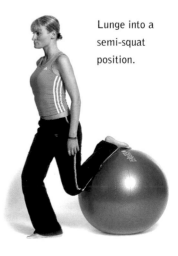

Lunge into a semi-squat position.

Side Lying Raise

Level: Basic

This exercise strengthens the inner thigh (adductors) and muscles, which control side bending of the lower spine (*quadratus lumborum*).

These are key stabilizing muscles, which work when the body has to change direction or bend to one side during sport.

Lie on your side on the exercise mat, place a smaller exercise ball between your feet.

Tighten the lower abdominal muscles and keeping your spine straight, slowly lift both feet from the floor. Hold for a few seconds then lower your feet back to the floor.

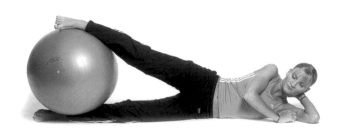

Place the ball between your ankles.

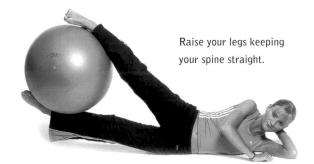

Raise your legs keeping your spine straight.

Squats

Level: Basic

Squatting is designed to strengthen the muscles at the front of the thigh (quadriceps). By adding the ball we create a need for the brain to maintain control of a moving object, while performing the exercise.

Stand with the ball between your lower back and the wall, with your feet shoulder width apart.

Maintaining a neutral spine position, squat no lower than 90 degrees, hold for a few seconds and return to a standing position. Your knees should be kept in alignment with your second toe.

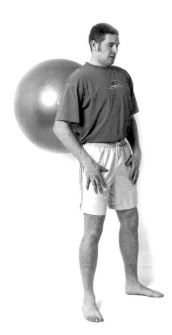

Stand with the ball between your lower back and the wall.

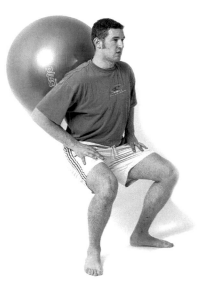

Squat no lower than 90 degrees.

Pushing Ball in Pairs

Level: Basic

Coordination and control of the lower limbs are the key elements to this exercise. Working in pairs or groups of three or four turns this into a fun team building activity.

Lie on your back on the floor or exercise mat with the ball between both pairs of feet. Tighten the lower abdominal muscles.

The ball is moved toward one person, then the other, without it touching the floor.

Place the ball between both pairs of feet.

The lower limbs should be creating the movement and control. Ensure the spine does not arch from the floor.

Offering differing amounts of resistance can make this exercise more difficult.

One person pushes, the other guides and controls.

Coordination in Pairs

Level: Basic

A greater degree of coordination is required to perform this exercise.

The brain now has to concentrate on moving and controlling the object, while also mimicking a running action.

Lie on the floor or exercise mats and place the ball between both pairs of feet.

Tighten the lower abdominal muscles and ensure the spine does not arch from the floor.

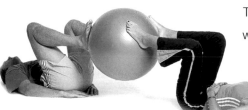

Place the ball between both pairs of feet.

Alternately push the ball toward each other in a slow running action, each partner changing legs each time the ball comes toward them.

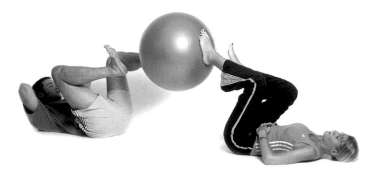

Control the ball using a slow running action.

Intermediate Exercises

Intermediate Double Leg Lifts

Level: Intermediate

This exercise may seem difficult at first until core stability improves, but practice is the key in order for the brain and muscle groups to act together. The muscles which flex the hip have to lift the lower limbs from the floor and hold them in free space.

Sit on the ball with your spine in a neutral position, tighten the lower abdominal muscles, and leaning very slightly backward, lift both feet a few inches from the floor.

Hold for a few seconds and return to the start position.

Your arms can be held out in front at chest height to assist with stability.

Soon you'll be able to lift the feet further from the floor without losing balance.

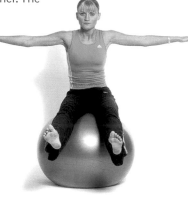

Sit on the ball with your feet shoulder width apart

Lean slightly backward lifting your feet from the floor.

Intermediate Leg Lifts

Level: Intermediate

Adding ankle weights to this exercise will strengthen the muscles in the leg as they lift against gravity.

Sit on the ball with your feet shoulder width apart, wearing ankle weights, and your arms relaxed by your side or crossed over your chest.

Tighten the lower abdominal muscles and slowly lift your right leg from the floor, extending at the knee to make it as straight as possible, hold for a few seconds, and slowly return to the start position. Repeat using the other leg. Do not lift the leg higher than your pelvis.

Remember to keep your spine straight, stomach muscles tight, and the ball as still as possible.

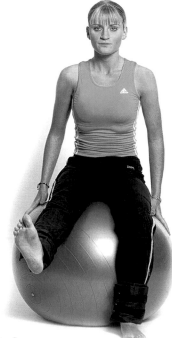

Flex your hip to lift the extended leg from the floor.

Intermediate Hamstring Curls

Level: Intermediate

By lifting one leg from the ball, the basic hamstring curl is adapted so that all the control and strength is coming from one side of the body only.

Lie on the floor or exercise mat with your heels on the ball and tighten the lower abdominal muscles. Lift one leg clear from the ball and extend. Using the other leg, slowly bring the ball toward the buttocks by tightening the hamstring muscles at the back of the thigh. Hold for a few seconds and extend your leg back to the start position. Change legs and repeat. The spine should not arch away from the floor during this exercise.

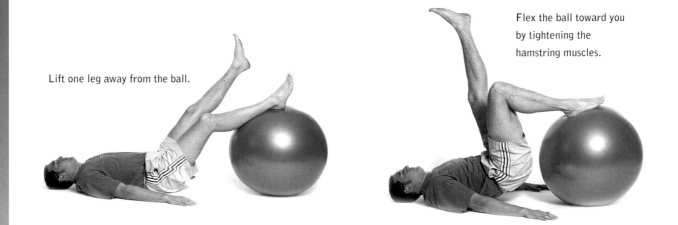

Lift one leg away from the ball.

Flex the ball toward you by tightening the hamstring muscles.

Hamstring Curl With Weights

Level: Intermediate

This exercise is performed exactly the same way as you would in the gym, but with the added instability of using the ball as the bench.

Wearing ankle weights, lie on the ball so that the ball is under your thighs.

Use your hands on the floor to offer stability and keeping a neutral spine position, flex the right ankle up toward your right buttock.

Hold for a few seconds and slowly return your leg to a horizontal position.

Change legs after the required number of repetitions.

Flex your ankle up toward your buttocks.

Hamstrings in Pairs

Level: Intermediate

This is a fun way to stretch the hamstring muscles and improve coordination.

Sit facing each other on the floor or exercise mat with the ball in the middle. Position your feet either side of the ball touching toes with your partner.

Both partners sit upright and tighten the lower abdominal muscles, placing their hands on top of the ball.

Flexing from the hips as though a steel rod was placed in the spine, slowly push the ball forward toward your partner, hold for a few seconds and reverse the position so that your partner is pushing the ball.

When this becomes too easy, simply move further way from each other.

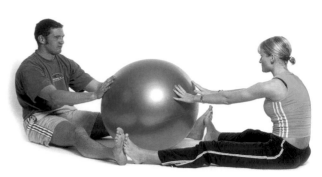

Sit facing each other with the ball in the middle.

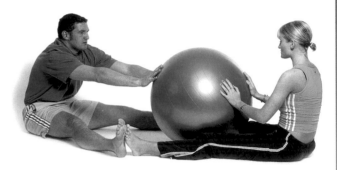

Lean forward as you push the ball from one to the other.

Intermediate Bridge

Level: Intermediate

Although this exercise is featured in the "Core Stability" section, it is also a great activity for strengthening the hamstring and calf muscles.

Lie on the floor or exercise mat with your feet placed flat on the ball and your arms by your sides. Tighten the lower abdominal muscles.

Lift your pelvis from the floor by using the hamstring and gluteal muscles until your body is in a diagonal position from your feet to your shoulders. (Do not cheat by using your arms to push your body upward!)

Hold for a few seconds and return to the start position.

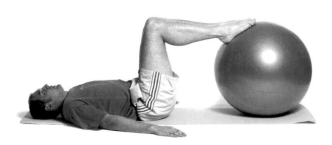

Start with your spine in neutral with your feet on the ball.

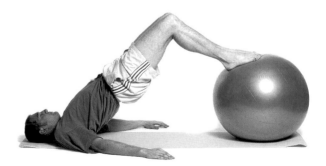

Lift your pelvis using the gluteal and hamstring muscles.

Intermediate Single Hip Flexion

Level: Intermediate

With one leg raised from the ball, the body's center of gravity is changed. The hip flexors in the remaining leg now have to work twice as hard to pull the ball toward your chest.

Lie with the ball under your stomach and roll forward until the ball is under your shins. Tighten the lower abdominal muscles and maintain a neutral alignment of the spine. Lift one leg clear from the ball and hold in this position. Slowly bring the ball toward your chest using the remaining leg ensuring that the lower spine is not allowed to sag or arch.

Return to the start position and repeat.

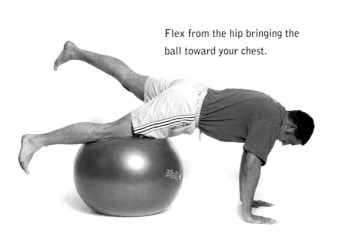

Flex from the hip bringing the ball toward your chest.

Roll forward until the ball is under your shins.

Single Leg Squats

Level: Intermediate

Here, the quadriceps in one leg are being asked to take your whole body weight while controlling movement from the ball.

Stand with the ball between your lower back and the wall, feet shoulder width apart. Maintaining a neutral spine, flex one leg at the hip and knee to lift the foot from the floor. Squat on the other leg no lower than 90 degrees, hold for a few seconds, and return to the standing position. Repeat using the other leg.

Remember that your hips and knees should be kept in alignment with your second toe.

Squat no lower than 90 degrees.

Lift one leg away from the floor.

Stability Cushion Squats

Level: Intermediate

During this squat exercise, the brain and muscles have to concentrate on balance as well as controlling the movement of the ball behind the body.

Stand with the ball between your lower back and the wall, feet on a stability cushion, shoulder width apart.

Maintaining a neutral spine position, squat no lower than 90 degrees, hold for a few seconds, and return to a standing position. Your knees should be kept in alignment with your second toe.

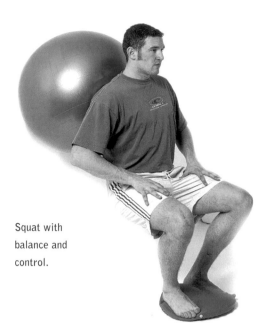

Squat with balance and control.

Piriformis

Level: Intermediate

The piriformis is a very small muscle that lies deep underneath the gluteals and is attached to the pelvis and top of the leg. Its job is to turn out the thigh and stop the knee from hanging inward.

Frequently, this muscle becomes over tense, leading to lack of mobility in the hip and in some cases compressing the sciatic nerve which runs under or through it, resulting in pain in the lower back and down the leg (sciatica), often mistaken for disc problems.

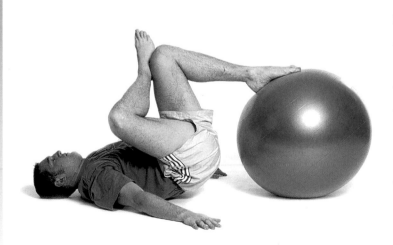

Flex the ball toward you, feeling the pull in the right buttock.

Lie on the floor or exercise mat with your left heel on the ball. Bring your right leg up to rest the ankle across your left knee.

Tighten the lower abdominal muscles and using the left foot, pull the ball toward your pelvis so that a pull is felt in the gluteal muscles of the right side.

Hold for 15 seconds, keeping the ball as steady as possible and return to the start position. Repeat using the opposite leg.

Limit this exercise to four repetitions on each side.

Intermediate Lunge

Level: Intermediate

Once you are confident with the basic lunge exercise, practice sports specific skills such as throwing and catching a ball, hitting a tennis or squash ball against a wall, or just use your imagination.

Try as a team skill activity to improve balance and coordination.

Stand facing a partner with the ball under the right shin. Slightly bend the left leg.

Maintaining a neutral spine, lunge forward so that left leg is in a squat position and the right leg is slightly extended on the ball.

In this position, throw a medicine ball to a partner a number of times. Return to the start position and repeat with the other leg. Do not allow the spine to arch backward during this exercise.

Try throwing and catching a medicine ball

Single Leg Squat with Cushion

Level: Intermediate

Stand with the ball between your lower back and the wall and your feet on a stability cushion, shoulder width apart. Lift one leg flexing at the hip and knee at 90 degrees.

Maintaining a neutral spine position, squat on the other leg no lower than 90 degrees, hold for a few seconds and return to a standing position. Your knees should be kept in alignment with the second toe.

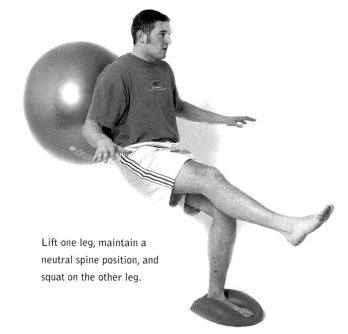

Lift one leg, maintain a neutral spine position, and squat on the other leg.

Advanced Exercises

Advanced Reverse Bridge

Level: Advanced

Squeezing the stability cushions between your thighs during this exercise encourages the inner thigh muscles (adductors) to work in harmony with the core stabilizing muscles. A discipline that is often required when side stepping as in tennis and squash.

With the ball positioned under your shoulders and the stability cushion placed between your knees, cross your arms over your chest and tighten your lower abdominal muscles. Squeeze the thigh muscles together as firmly as you can without arching or dipping the lumbar spine. Hold this squeeze for a few seconds, release and repeat.

Advanced Hip Extension

Level: Advanced

Lifting the leg while wearing ankle weights increases strength in the gluteal, hamstring, and lower leg muscle groups.

Put on ankle weights and position yourself over the ball so that it is under the thighs and pelvis.

Flex your right leg at the knee to 90 degrees and then push the foot upward to lift the thigh away from the ball by extending the hip as far as you can go.

Hold for a few seconds, slowly return to the start position and repeat with the other leg.

Maintain a neutral alignment of the spine throughout this exercise.

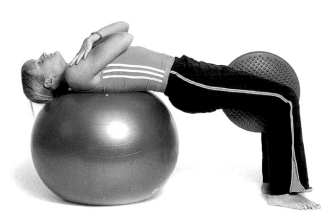

Maintain a neutral spine position and squeeze the thighs together.

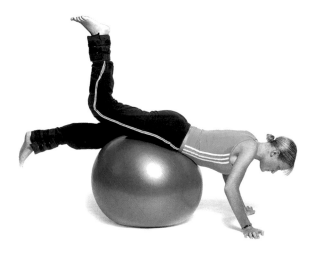

Flex at the knee 90 degrees and push upward.

Advanced Squats
Level: Advanced

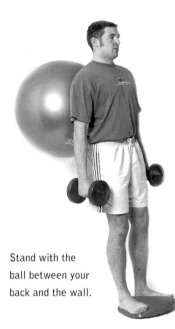

Stand with the ball between your back and the wall.

Squatting while holding dumbbells increases the weight load on the quadriceps, helping to strengthen the muscles.

Hold dumbbells in both hands by your sides. Stand with the ball between your lower back and the wall, feet on a stability cushion, shoulder width apart.

Maintaining neutral spine, squat no lower than 90 degrees, hold for a few seconds and slowly return to a standing position. Your knees should be kept in alignment with the second toe.

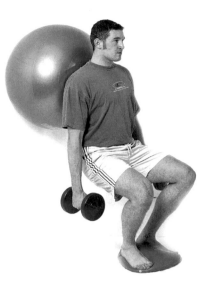

Squat and hold for a few seconds before returning to a standing position.

Squatting in Pairs
Level: Advanced

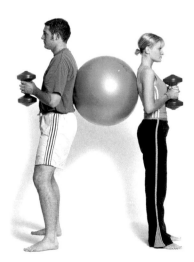

Start back to back with the ball in between.

This is a great team building exercise. Increased coordination is required to keep the ball level and to maintain balance and alignment.

Stand back to back with the ball between your lower backs and feet shoulder width apart.

Maintaining a neutral spine position and equal speed, both squat no lower than 90 degrees, controlling the ball in a central position. Hold for a few seconds and slowly both return to a standing position.

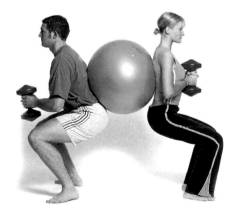

Control alignment and balance as you squat.

Your knees should be kept in alignment with the second toe.

You can hold dumbbells or stand on stability cushions to make the exercise more difficult.

Lateral Squat

Level: Advanced

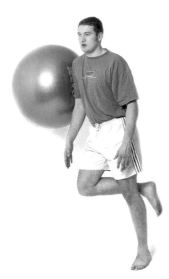

Stand at a 45-degree angle with the ball between the wall and your right side.

Squatting at an angle builds specific strength needed for sports where the body is moving to the side, changing direction quickly, or running while keeping the body low, such as in rugby or American football.

Stand at a 45 degree angle with the ball between the wall and your right side at elbow height. Lift your inside leg from the floor and squat on the outside leg, no lower than 90 degrees. Hold for a few seconds then use the leg muscles to slowly extend back to the start position. Keep your hips, shoulders and spine in alignment throughout this exercise.

Repeat the exercise using the inside leg, then turn around and repeat with ball against the left side.

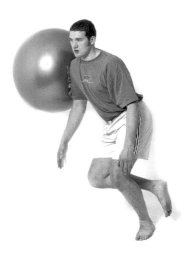

Lift your inside leg from the floor and squat on your outside leg.

Advanced Double Leg Lifts

Level: Advanced

The addition of ankle weights in this exercise changes the body's center of gravity and makes lifting the legs from the floor more difficult.

Wear ankle weights and sit on the ball with your spine in a neutral position. Tighten the lower abdominal muscles and lean very slightly backward. Lift both feet a few inches from the floor. Hold for a few seconds and return to the start position.

Your arms can be held out in front at chest height to assist with stability.

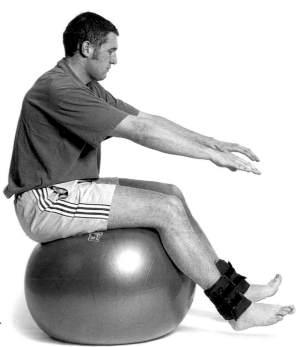

Use ankle weights to make lifting the legs more difficult.

Advanced Lunge

Level: Advanced

Strength is enhanced in the quadriceps, pelvis, and leg muscles, while the stabilizing muscle groups are concentrating on postural alignment and balance.

Stand with the ball under the right shin and hold a medicine ball or dumbbells out at chest height. Slightly bend the left leg.

Maintaining a neutral spine, lunge forward so that left leg is in a squat position and right leg is extended on the ball. Hold for two seconds and return to the start position and repeat with the other leg. Do not allow the spine to arch backward during this exercise.

Advance this exercise by holding one dumbbell or the medicine ball out at chest height and as you lunge forward, rotate the upper torso to one side (as if passing the ball to someone coming from behind).

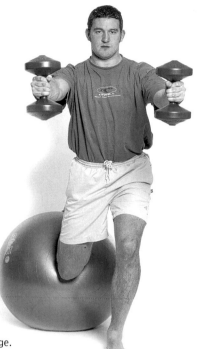

Use weights or a medicine ball to add sports specific skills to the lunge.

Running in Pairs

Level: Advanced

Many of the stabilizing muscle groups are at work to control balance and coordination while upper torso muscle groups are actively engaged holding the dumbbells.

Lie on mats and place the ball between both pairs of feet. Each partner holds a medicine ball or dumbbells out from the body at chest level.

Tighten the lower abdominal muscles and ensure the spine does not arch from the floor

Alternately push the ball toward each other in a running action, each partner changing legs each time the ball comes toward them.

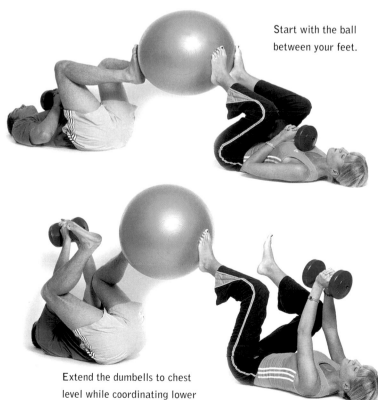

Start with the ball between your feet.

Extend the dumbells to chest level while coordinating lower limb movement of the ball.

109

Senior Citizens

Exercise is just as important, if not more so, as we get older. Research shows that moderate exercise improves bone strength and heart and lung function in the older population.

Using the exercise ball allows those, who do not want to take on rigorous gym regimes to exercise at their own pace in their own time with very little cost. It also adds an element of fun, while encouraging the other important aspects of coordination and balance.

In this section a Physio Roll* has been introduced, which is of similar material to the ball but is shaped like a peanut. This shape means that the roll can only move in one plane of motion, reducing the risk of falls, and increasing confidence for those who may find the ball too unstable.

Senior citizens should not feel that they are just limited to this basic section of the book as many are quite capable of carrying out the activities even to intermediate and advanced level. But it is always wise to check with your doctor or physician to ensure you do not put yourself at risk of injury.

* Registered trademark of Ledraplastic Spa. Italy

Abdominals

Level: Basic

As we get older, the strength of the abdominal muscles is even more important to counteract the narrowing of the disc spaces of the lower back, which result in stiffness, lack of mobility, and pain.

Sit on the Physio Roll or ball with feet shoulder width apart.

Hold your arms out in front to maintain balance and gently lean backward until the lower abdominal muscles tighten. Try to hold for a few seconds and slowly return to the start position.

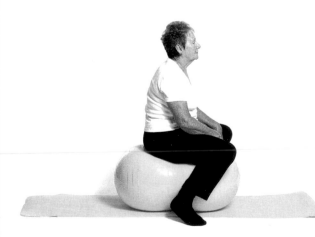

Sit with your spine as straight as possible.

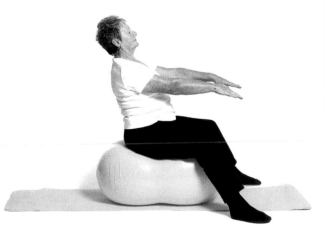

Lean slightly backward until your stomach muscles tighten.

Side Extension

Level: Basic

Maintaining flexibility of the spine is important if we are to avoid the muscle strain and backache associated with stiffness and poor mobility.

Sit on a ball with your feet shoulder width apart. Tighten the stomach muscles and raise the right arm.

Slowly reach down the side of the ball with the left hand flexing the spine sideways, hold for a few seconds and slowly return to the start position. Repeat on the other side.

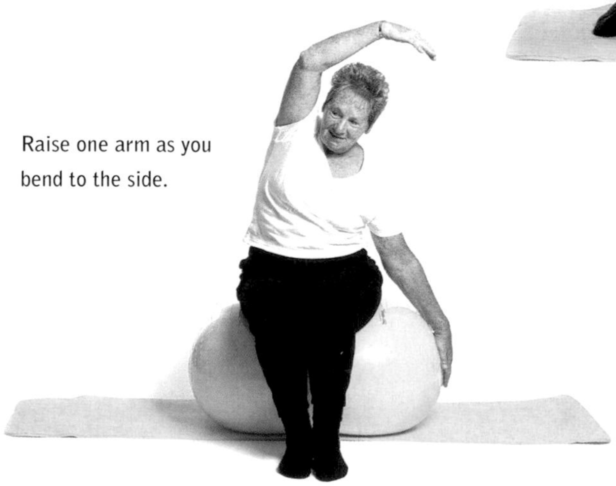

Spinal Flexion

Level: Basic

The spine compresses under the weight of our bodies as we go about our daily activities, especially if we are seated for long periods.

Flexing the spine forward over the ball is an ideal way to allow gravity to apply natural traction, opening out the vertebrae and stretching the muscles.

Kneel on a cushion or exercise mat with the ball under your chest.

Gently push forward until the ball is under your stomach and your spine is arched.

Allow your arms to hang down and slowly roll backward and foward while relaxing over the ball.

Do this exercise for about 30 seconds.

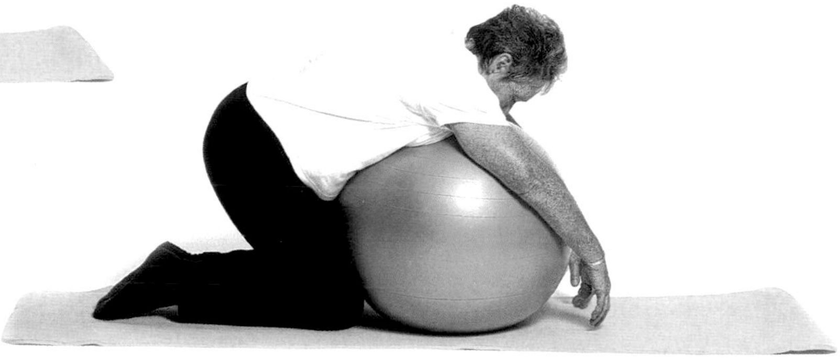

Sit with your feet shoulder width apart.

Relax over the ball to open out the spine.

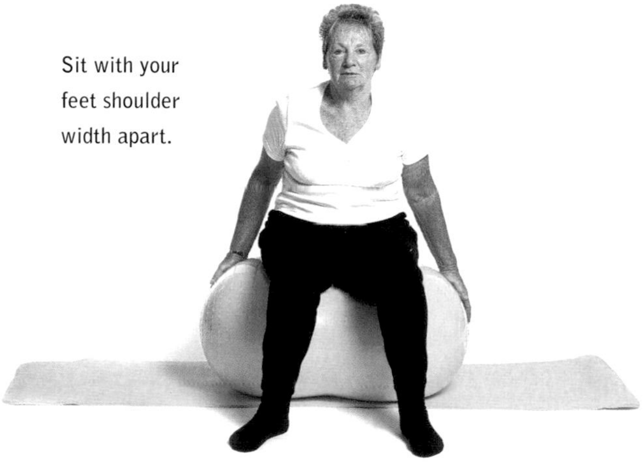

Raise one arm as you bend to the side.

Side Flexion

Level: Basic

Keeping the muscles of the lower back and side toned helps us to carry out every day activities without risking pulled muscles.

Sit on the ball with your feet placed shoulder width apart. Tighten the lower abdominal muscles and place your hands by your sides touching the ball. Slowly reach down to one side as far as you can go, you should feel the muscles in your side tighten.

Hold for a few seconds and slowly return to the start position. Repeat using the opposite side.

Side Rotation

Level: Basic

Turning the body from one side to another requires the bones of the spine (vertebrae) to rotate. Many muscles activate and control this rotation and regular exercise is needed to keep these strong and supple.

Sit on the ball with your feet shoulder width apart. Tighten the lower abdominal muscles.

Bring your arms to chest level. From this position gently rotate your upper body round to the right as far as is comfortable, keeping the pelvis level on the ball and then slowly return to face the middle. Repeat the rotation to the left.

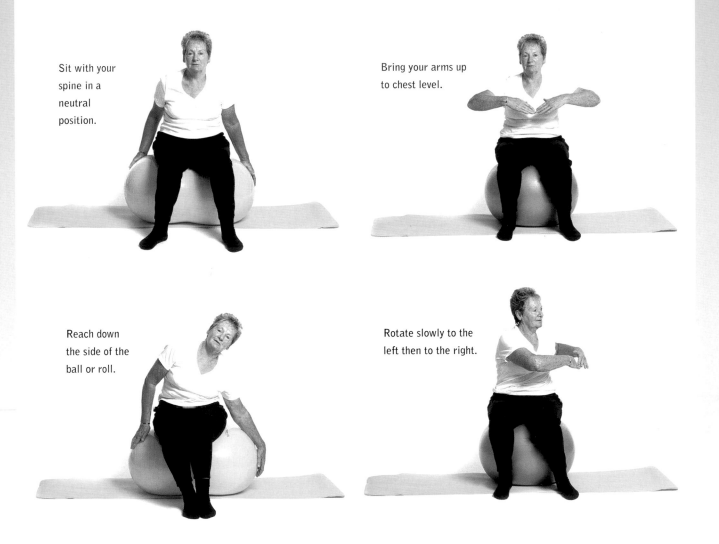

Sit with your spine in a neutral position.

Bring your arms up to chest level.

Reach down the side of the ball or roll.

Rotate slowly to the left then to the right.

Pelvic Rotation

Level: Basic

As we get older our sense of balance may not be what it once was, making it easier for us to slip and fall.

This exercise helps to strengthen the muscles of the legs and lower spine, while improving flexibility in the pelvis.

Sit on the ball with your feet shoulder width apart and your hands placed at either side, touching the ball or held out to the side to assist with balance.

Tighten the lower abdominal muscles and use your pelvis to slowly rotate the ball in small clockwise and anticlockwise circles.

Ensure the spine is kept straight throughout. If you are finding this difficult, try making smaller circles.

Pelvic Tilts

Level: Basic

Our gluteal (buttock) muscles play a very important role in the movements of the hip and upper leg. By pushing our pelvis from one side to the other, we cause these muscles to contract (tighten), making them stronger and more efficient.

Sit on the ball with your feet shoulder width apart and your arms on either side touching the ball.

Tighten the lower abdominal muscles and tighten the gluteal muscles to push the pelvis to the left. Hold for a few seconds and return to the start position. Repeat the tilt to the opposite side.

Ensure your spine stays straight and your feet are kept firmly on the floor throughout this exercise.

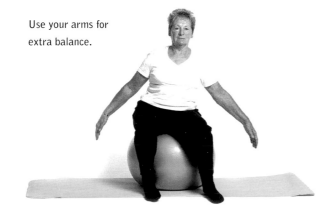

Use your arms for extra balance.

Sit on the ball with your spine in a neutral position.

Rotate the ball in small circles using your pelvis.

Use the buttock muscles to push the pelvis from one side to another.

Hip Flexion

Level: Basic

The hip flexors are also responsible for the stability of the lower back. If these muscles are tight or out of balance, the lower back often becomes painful and hip mobility can be reduced.

Sit on the ball with your feet shoulder width apart and your arms by your sides touching the ball.

Slowly lift one leg up toward your chest, keeping the ball steady. Hold for a few seconds and return to the start position. Repeat with the other leg.

Keep your back as straight as possible throughout.

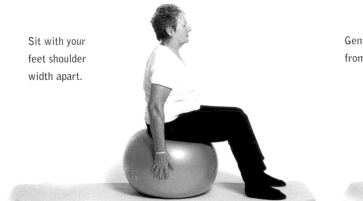

Sit with your feet shoulder width apart.

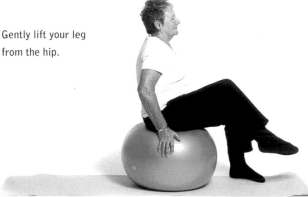

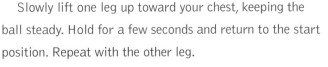

Gently lift your leg from the hip.

Leg Strengthening

Level: Basic

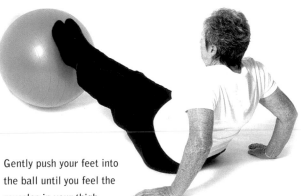

Gently push your feet into the ball until you feel the muscles in your thigh tighten.

The muscles in front of the thigh (quadriceps) need to be kept active. A weakness in this muscle group leads to difficulty when lifting the thigh and straightening the knee.

Place the ball against the wall and sit on the floor or a chair facing the wall. Place one or both feet on the ball.

Keeping the spine straight and holding onto the chair arms for support if needed, slowly push your feet into the ball until you feel the muscles in the thigh tighten. Hold for a few seconds and repeat.

Change to the other foot if you are using only one foot at a time.

Adductor Strengthening

Level: Basic

The inner thigh muscles (adductors) form part of the stabilizing group for the pelvis and lower limbs. It is this muscle group which "pulls up" or tightens to stop a foot slipping out to the side.

Sit on the floor or in a chair and place the exercise ball between your knees and lower legs.

Slowly squeeze the knees together so that the insides of the thighs tighten. Hold for a few seconds, release, and repeat.

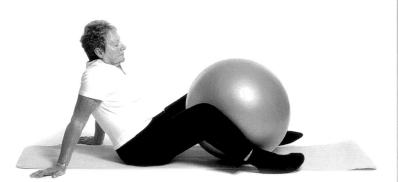

Gently squeeze your knees together.

Knee Extension with Band

Level: Basic

This exercise will strengthen the muscles at the front of the thigh, helping to stabilize the knee joint.

Sit on the ball with your feet shoulder width apart, place the resistance band around both feet.

Gently lift one leg forward pulling on the band as far as you can, hold for a few seconds and return to the start position. Repeat as many times as necessary, then change feet and repeat with the opposite leg.

Remember not to let your back arch or sag during this exercise.

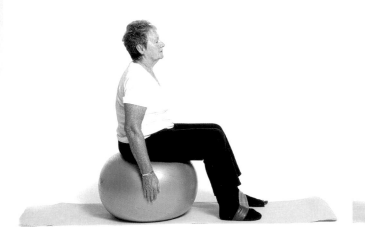

Place a band around both feet.

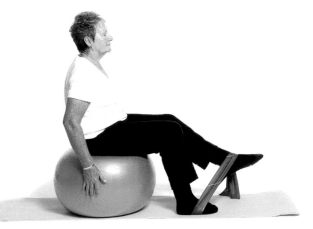

Lift one leg, pulling the band as far as you can.

Side Toe Touches

Level: Basic

This exercise helps to work the muscles on the inside and outside of the thigh, as well as improving balance in the lower back muscles.

Sit on the ball with your feet shoulder width apart and your arms placed on either side touching the ball.

Alternately touch your toes out to the side trying to keep the ball steady at the same time.

Keep your pelvis level and your spine straight, the movement should only come from the legs.

Start slowly at first as the object of this exercise is to keep the ball as still as possible throughout.

Toe Touches

Level: Basic

Touching the toes out to the front will help to strengthen the muscles in the middle of the thigh and the hip.

Sit on the ball with your feet shoulder width apart and your hands at either side touching the ball.

Touch each toe on the ground in front of you, keeping the ball as steady as possible.

Remember to start slowly as the object of the exercise is to keep the ball from moving around.

You may find it helpful to hold the arms out in front for balance.

Sit with your feet shoulder width apart.

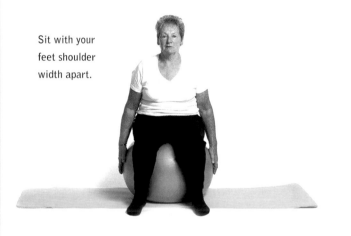

Sit with your spine straight.

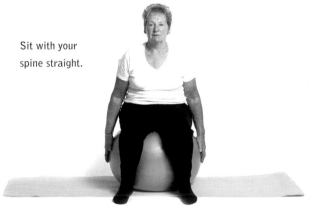

Touch your toe out to the side as far as you can.

Touch each toe out in front.

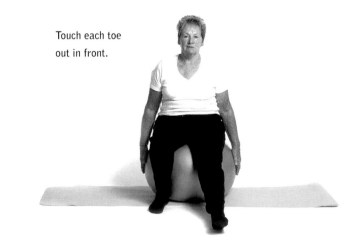

Single Leg Lifts

Level: Basic

Lifting and extending the leg from the floor strengthens not only the leg muscles, but those of the back and abdomen.

Sit on the ball with your feet shoulder width apart and your hands on either side touching the ball.

Slowly lift the left leg from the floor and straighten as far as you can at the knee, hold for a few seconds and slowly return to the start position. Repeat using the other leg.

Remember to keep the stomach muscles tight and the ball as still as possible.

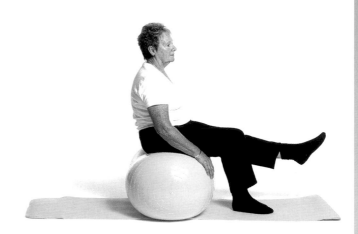

Lift your leg and extend the knee as straight as possible.

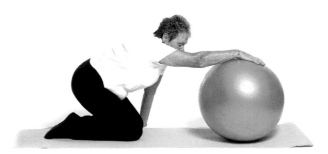

Kneel or sit with one hand resting on the ball.

Kneeling Shoulder Mobility

Level: Basic

Moving the ball in an arc from head to toe maintains mobility in the shoulder joint.

If this joint or the muscles around it become stiff, simple things like putting on a jacket or even brushing your hair can become very difficult.

Kneel on a cushion or exercise mat in a position you find comfortable with the ball under one hand.

Keeping your hand on the ball, slowly draw a semicircle from your head down toward your feet and back again.

Only use the shoulder to move the ball and do not bend at the side or hips.

If kneeling is difficult, try this exercise in a seated position on the floor instead and move the ball from your front to your side.

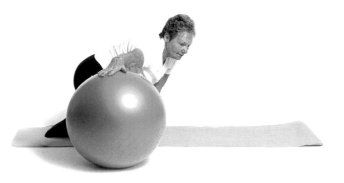

Use your shoulder to move the ball from head to toe.

Shoulder Rotation

Level: Basic

The muscles at the back of your shoulder can become weakened, resulting in poor movement and even pain.

This exercise strengthens these muscles and helps to improve posture.

Sit on the ball, place the resistance band under your left foot, and hold it in your right hand.

Start with your arm relaxed in front of you, then gently pull the band outward and backward as far as you can. Hold for a few seconds, release and repeat.

Change the exercise band to the right foot and repeat with the left arm.

Remember to keep the stomach muscles tightened and your spine as straight as possible.

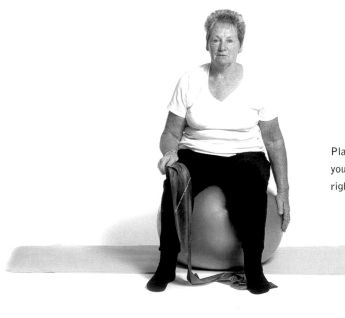

Place the resistance band under your left foot and hold it in your right hand.

Gently pull your arm out and up as far as you can.

Shoulder Abduction

Level: Basic

This exercise will help to strengthen the muscles that lift your arm to the side and improve stability of the shoulder joint.

Sit on the ball, place the resistance band under your right foot and hold it in your right hand.

Gently lift your right arm out to the side, raising it no higher than your shoulder. Hold for a few seconds and release. Change the exercise band to your left foot and repeat with your left arm.

Remember to keep the stomach muscles tightened and your spine straight.

Shoulder Extension

Level: Basic

The muscles in the front of the shoulder often become tight, restricting movement and in some cases, causing pain. By rolling the ball up the wall, these muscles are stretched, improving your range of movement.

Hold a ball against the wall at chest level. Keeping the spine straight, slowly roll the ball up the wall as far as you can, hold for a few seconds and bring back to the start position. If this is too easy, you can use one hand placed on the ball and the other behind your back alternating after a few repetitions.

The movement should only come from the shoulders. Do not allow the body to lean on the ball.

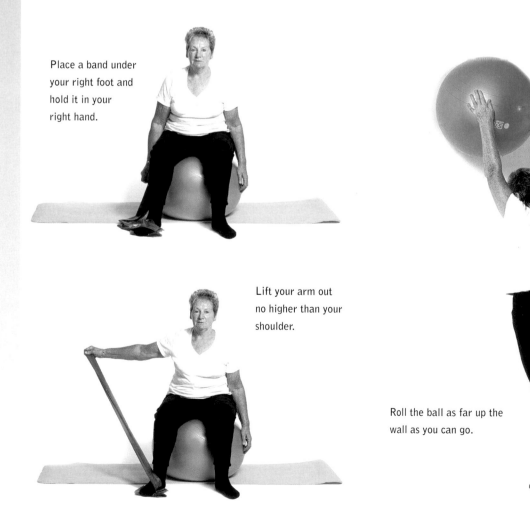

Place a band under your right foot and hold it in your right hand.

Lift your arm out no higher than your shoulder.

Roll the ball as far up the wall as you can go.

Antenatal and Postnatal

Use of the exercise ball is rapidly becoming popular for pregnant women and is employed widely in clinics and hospitals all over the world.

Many women, especially in the later stages of pregnancy, find that the ball is the only comfortable place to sit as it allows the pelvis to be level or very slightly higher than the knees. This position creates a better posture, leaving more room for the baby to move around, which results in less discomfort for the mother.

Exercise before the birth is important if the mother is to keep strong and healthy. However, this has to be kept very basic, mainly due to mum's shape inhibiting movement, but also for safety so that no strain is placed on the muscles of the abdomen. After birth, the pelvic muscles need to be strengthened. The ball is a great tool for improving the pelvic floor.

Mothers have also commented that sitting on the ball with the baby in your arms is very soothing for the child, as it allows gentle, relaxing movement.

Using the Physio Roll may also be an option for these exercises, as it will allow a little more stability than the ball, enabling mum to gain her confidence.

A pregnant woman should always seek medical advice before commencing any exercise and ensure that she checks with her doctor or midwife that the ball and exercises are suitable for her.

Recently, the exercise balls have also proved popular in the delivery room. During the birth of the baby, the ball provides support in the kneeling or squatting positions and can allow the mother to keep moving to ease the discomfort.

Your midwife can advise on the suitability of this application.

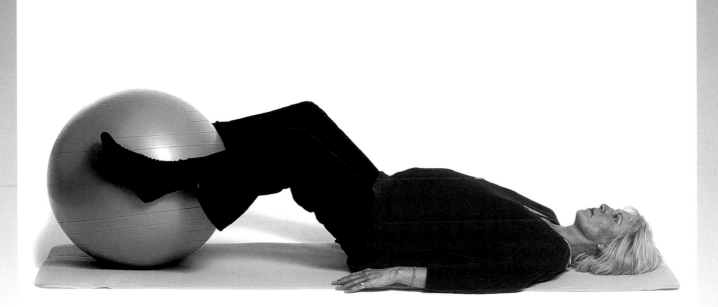

Sitting

Level: All

Not only is the ball suitable for antenatal and postnatal exercise to help keep the mother fit, but many pregnant women find it a more comfortable alternative to a chair, especially in the later stages.

Sitting on the ball creates good posture, allowing more room for the baby and making life more comfortable for the baby and mother. Because the pelvis is maintained in a position slightly higher than the knees, this creates an optimum position for the engagement of the baby's head toward the end of the last trimester.

When seated on the ball, the pelvis should be slightly higher than the knees and, just like the section in the front of the book on neutral alignment, the back should be as straight as possible. Your feet should be flat on the floor, shoulder width apart.

Babies do not always lie in the most comfortable position for the mother and by gently rotating and tilting the pelvis, an optimum comfortable position can usually be obtained.

Kneeling

Level: All

Kneeling or leaning over the ball can be a very comfortable position for most pregnant females.

Many babies lie in a posterior position (their back to the mother's back). This is heavy work on the mother often causing lower backache and general fatigue.

Leaning on the ball in this manner is not only comfortable for mum but can assist in turning the baby into a better position. Women often find this position very comfortable during labor.

Kneel on a pillow with the ball in front of you or supported against a wall or immovable object.

Rest your upper body on the ball in a position comfortable for you.

Drape a towel over the ball to make it more comfortable if you wish to rest this way for a period of time.

If needed, place a cushion or pillow between your heels and bottom for comfort.

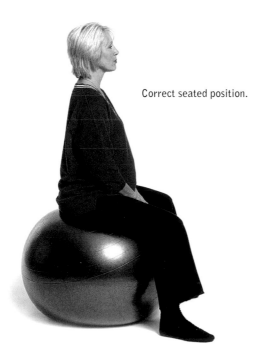

Correct seated position.

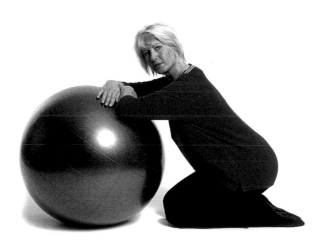

Kneeling position.

Pelvic Rotation

Level: All

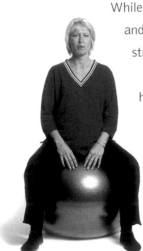

While rotating the ball gently, not only are you able to keep the pelvis and lower back mobile but this movement helps to maintain strength in the legs as they assist in movement and balance.

Sit on the ball with your feet shoulder width apart and your hands placed on either side touching the ball.

Use your pelvis to slowly rotate the ball in small clockwise and anticlockwise circles.

Ensure your spine is kept as straight as possible throughout. If this is difficult, then try making smaller circles.

Your feet should remain flat on the floor to maintain stability.

Sit with your feet shoulder width apart and your spine in neutral.

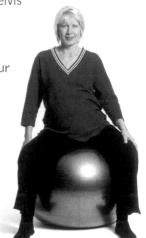

Rotate the pelvis gently in a clockwise or anticlockwise direction.

Pelvic Tilts

Level: All

Using your pelvis to move the ball helps to keep the lower back muscles mobile, while at the same time strengthening the core muscles, which the pregnant woman will need for delivery.

Sit with your feet shoulder width apart and your spine in a neutral position.

Sit on the ball with your feet shoulder width apart and your arms on either side touching the ball.

Use your pelvis to gently push the ball to the left and right alternately.

Ensure your spine stays as straight as possible and your feet are kept firmly on the floor throughout this exercise.

Tilt your pelvis gently from side to side.

Side Flexion

Level: All

This exercise mobilizes and strengthens the sacrospinalis muscle ,which runs the full length of the spine from the pelvis to the base of the skull, attaching to each vertebrae and at various points into the ribs.

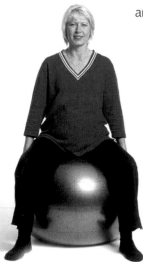

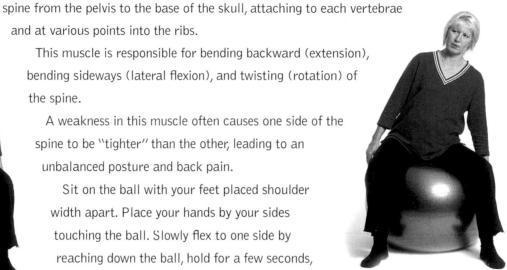

This muscle is responsible for bending backward (extension), bending sideways (lateral flexion), and twisting (rotation) of the spine.

A weakness in this muscle often causes one side of the spine to be "tighter" than the other, leading to an unbalanced posture and back pain.

Sit on the ball with your feet placed shoulder width apart. Place your hands by your sides touching the ball. Slowly flex to one side by reaching down the ball, hold for a few seconds, and return to the start position. Repeat using the opposite side. Try not to arch or hollow the spine during this exercise.

Sit with your feet shoulder width apart.

Flex gently to either side

Toe Touches

Level: All

What may seem like a very simple exercise uses many muscle groups in the pelvis and legs. While doing this, the spine is also still having to work at stabilizing the ball, which strengthens the smaller, deeper muscles of the spine (multifidus), responsible for posture and strength.

Sit on the ball with your feet shoulder width apart and your hands at either side touching the ball.

Alternately touch each toe on the ground in front of you keeping the ball as steady as possible.

Remember to start slowly as the object of the exercise is to keep the ball from moving around.

You may find it helpful to hold your arms out in front for balance.

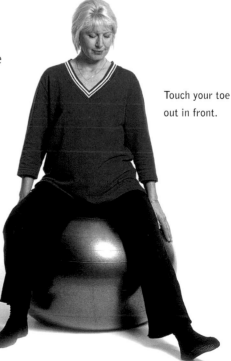

Touch your toe out in front.

Lateral Extension

Level: All

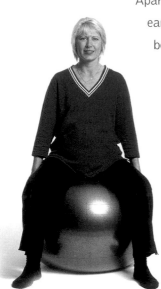

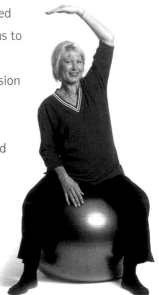

Apart from stretching the larger sacrospinalis muscle mentioned earlier, this exercise also stretches the muscle, which allows us to bend sideways (lateral flexion) and assists the diaphragm.

Mobility in this muscle reduces backache and eases tension on the diaphragm allowing the mother to breathe more efficiently.

Sit on the ball with your feet shoulder width apart and your arms by your sides touching the ball.

Keeping your pelvis level, raise your left arm up and extend it over your head, flexing the spine gently to the right side.

Try not to arch or hollow your back during this exercise.

Start in a seated position.

Gently extend over to side.

Pelvic Raises

Level: All

A more gentle version of the bridge position works the buttock (gluteal), back of thigh (hamstring), and thigh (quadriceps) muscle groups to provide a light, strengthening action.

During this exercise, the pelvic stabilizers are also activated, which makes it an ideal exercise for strengthening the pelvis muscles after giving birth.

Lie on the exercise mat with your feet on the ball, place your arms by your sides to add stability.

By pressing the legs into the ball and tightening the gluteal muscles, raise your pelvis from the floor about 4in. (10cm), hold for a few seconds, and then gently lower back down to the start position.

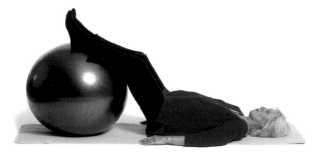

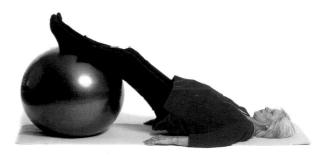

Rest your legs on the ball and keep your arms relaxed by your side.

Raise your pelvis gently from the floor.

Single Leg Raises

Level: All

The natural action of gravity on the inner thigh muscles (adductors) of the leg lifted from the ball provides a strengthening action.

Many women find that this muscle group aches after giving birth (especially if they have been laid on their back with their feet in stirrups). Strengthening them prior to the event should help alleviate some of the strain.

Lie on the exercise mat with your feet on ball and your arms placed by your sides.

Lift your right leg from the ball and turn the leg from the hip, so that your toes are facing slightly to the side.

Hold the position for a few seconds, then lower back to the ball and repeat with the other leg.

Knee Flexion

Level: All

The expectant mother is able to exercise and strengthen the muscles at the back of the thigh (hamstrings), while in a safe and stable position.

This exercise also helps to strengthen the hip flexor muscles at the front of the pelvis, which play an important part in pelvic stability.

Lie on the exercise mat with your feet on the ball and your arms placed by your sides.

Using your legs, gently roll the ball toward the buttocks. You should feel the muscles tighten at the back of the thigh. Hold for a few seconds then push away again. Do not allow the muscles to cramp during this exercise.

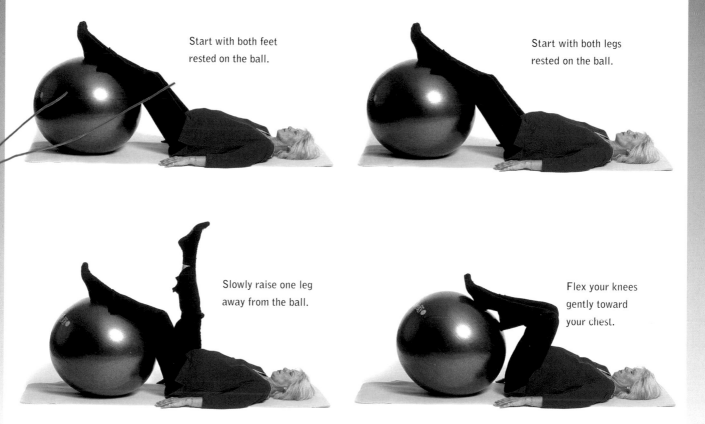

Start with both feet rested on the ball.

Start with both legs rested on the ball.

Slowly raise one leg away from the ball.

Flex your knees gently toward your chest.

Lumbar Rotation

Level: All

Gentle rotation of the lower spine (lumbar vertebrae) helps keep the lower back mobile. This is a great exercise for easing lower backache caused by being seated or standing in one position for great lengths of time.

Lay on the exercise mat with your feet on the ball shoulder width apart and your arms in a relaxed position by your side. Slowly rotate the ball from left to right using your feet, causing a gentle rotation of the lower spine.

Be careful not to rotate too far as this puts pressure on your abdominal muscles. You should feel no strain when doing this exercise, it should be quite relaxing.

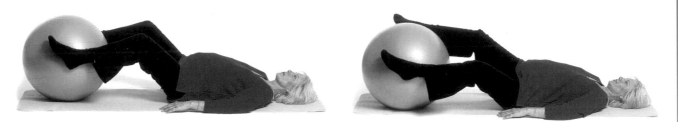

Place your feet on the ball at either side.   Gently rotate from side to side.

Leg Strengthening

Level: All

Pushing the feet into the ball strengthens the muscles at the front of the thigh (quadriceps).

This exercise is very useful if the mother is used to working out in the gym and does not want to lose the muscle tone in this area.

Position the ball against a wall. Lay on the exercise mat with your feet on the ball shoulder width apart and your arms in a relaxed position by your side. Gently push your feet into the ball to feel the muscles tighten in the thigh.

Hold for a few seconds and repeat. For comfort, this exercise can also be done seated on a chair instead of on the floor. You should feel no strain in the abdominal muscles during this exercise.

Slowly and steadily push your feet into the ball.

References

Bunton E.E., Pitney W.A., Kane A.W., et al: *The role of limb torque, muscle action and proprioception during closed kinetic chain rehabilitation of the lower extremity.* J Ath Training, 1993.

Caraffa A., Cerulli G., Projetti M., et al: *Prevention of anterior cruciate ligament injuries in soccer: a prospective controlled study of proprioceptive training.* Knee Surg Sport Traumatol Arthrosc, 1996.

Hides J.A., Richardson C.A., Jull G.A.: "Multifidus muscle recovery is not automatic after resolution of acute first episode low back pain" from *Spine,* Volume 21, 1996.

Norris C.: "Spinal stabilisation: Parts 1 to 5" from *Physiotherapy,* Volume 81, 1995.

Fitzgerald D.: "Using the gymnastic ball" from *Physiotherapy in Sport,* Volume 20, No.1, 1997.

Schutte M.J., Happel L.T.: "Joint innervation in joint injury." from *Clinical Sports Med,* 1990.

Glencross D., Thornton E.: "Position sense following joint injury." from *J Sports Med Physical Fitness,* 1991.

Lephart S.: "Re-establishing proprioception, kinaesthesia, joint position sense, and neuromuscular control in rehabilitation" from Prentice W.E. (ed): *Rehabilitation Techniques in Sports Medicine,* CV Mosby, St Louis, 1994.

Index